Preventing Alcohol and Tobacco Problems Volume 1

The Addiction Market: Consumption, Production and Policy Development

Edited by

ALAN MAYNARD
Professor of Economics, University of York

and

PHILIP TETHER
Senior Research Fellow, University of Hull

Avebury

Aldershot · Brookfield USA · Hong Kong · Singapore · Sydney

Published by

Avebury

Gower Publishing Company Limited
Gower House
Croft Road
Aldershot
Hants GU11 3HR
England

Gower Publishing Company,
Old Post Road,
Brookfield,
Vermont 05036,
U.S.A.

Printed and Bound in Great Britain by
Athenaeum Press Ltd., Newcastle upon Tyne.

ISBN 0 566 05701 8

Laserset by Computype, 241 Hull Road, York YO1 3LA

Contents

List of tables and figures   vii

List of contributors   xi

Foreword   xii

Acknowledgements   xvi

Editors' introduction: *Alan Maynard and Philip Tether*   1

Chapter 1   Consumption and taxation trends: *Geoff Hardman and Alan Maynard*   8

Chapter 2   Modelling demand: *Christine Godfrey*   35

Chapter 3   Preventive health objectives and tax policy options: *Christine Godfrey and Larry Harrison*   54

Chapter 4   Tax policy: structure and process: *Larry Harrison and Philip Tether*   75

Chapter 5   Tax policy and budget decisions: *Wendy*   96
             Leedham and Christine Godfrey

Chapter 6   Alcohol and tobacco: the politics of prevention: 117
             Rob Baggott

Chapter 7   Industry and employment policy: department   133
             and group relations: *Philip Tether and Larry*
             Harrison

Chapter 8   Industry: structure, performance and policy: 151
             Mark Booth, Keith Hartley and Melanie Powell

Chapter 9   Prevention policy and the Scotch whisky   179
             industry: *Mark Booth and Ron Weir*

Chapter 10   Employment: *Christine Godfrey and Keith*   204
             Hartley

Contents of Volume 2   227

Addiction Research Centre Bibliography   229

Index   237

List of tables and figures

Table 1.1:	Consumer expenditure on alcoholic drinks and tobacco at constant 1980 prices: £ million	10
Table 1.2:	Product shares in the alcohol industry as percentages of the total alcoholic drink market	12
Table 1.3:	Expenditure on alcoholic drinks and tobacco as a percentage of total consumer expenditure	13
Table 1.4:	Consumption of alcoholic drink: quantities released for home consumption—million litres	14
Table 1.5:	Consumption per capita of pure alcohol (in litres per head of population aged 15 and over)—calendar year data	16
Table 1.6:	Consumption of tobacco products in the UK by numbers and weight	17
Table 1.7:	Average weekly cigarette consumption by current smokers by sex and age: Great Britain	18
Table 1.8:	Commodity price indices relative to 'all items'—1963=100	20
Table 1.9:	Purchasing power: price in relation to personal disposable income	21

Table 1.10a:	Minutes of work required to earn the price of a pint of draught beer	22
Table 1.10b:	Hours of work required to earn the price of a bottle of whisky	23
Table 1.10c:	Hours of work required to earn the price of a bottle of wine	24
Table 1.10d:	Minutes of work required to earn the price of 20 cigarettes	25
Table 1.11a:	Tobacco duty rates 1960-1988	27
Table 1.11b:	Alcohol duty rates 1960-1988	29
Table 1.12:	Revenue from alcoholic drink and tobacco	31
Table 2.1:	Price elasticity estimates	45
Table 2.2:	Income elasticity estimates	46
Table 2.3:	Own price and income elasticities of earlier studies	48
Table 2.4:	Price and income elasticities for wines and spirits (evaluated for 1980)	49
Table 3.1:	Effects of a 5% revalorisation, 1986	62
Table 3.2:	Illustrative consumption and revenue changes from various policies	64
Table 3.3:	Illustrative changes of tax policies designed to equate tax or price per unit alcohol	68
Table 3.4:	Commission proposals for harmonised excise rates	70
Table 5.1:	Types of parliamentary questions 1974-1987	102
Table 5.2:	Approval/disapproval of increased taxation on cigarettes	105
Table 5.3:	Annual changes in excise tax rates and retail prices, 1974- 78, (%)	106
Table 5.4:	Changes in the prices and tax incidence for typical products as a result of budgets, 1974-78	107
Table 5.5:	Annual changes in excise tax rates and retail prices, 1979- 1983, (%)	110
Table 5.6:	Changes in the prices and tax incidence for typical products as a result of budgets, 1979-83	110
Table 5.7:	Annual changes in excise tax rates and retail prices, 1984- 88, (%)	112
Table 5.8:	Changes in the prices and tax incidence for typical products as a result of budgets, 1984-88	112
Table 6.1:	Economic leverage of the alcohol and tobacco industry	124

Table 8.1:	The UK alcohol and tobacco industries	157
Table 8.2:	Output of UK alcohol and tobacco industries	160
Table 8.3:	UK alcohol and tobacco companies	163
Table 8.4:	Concentration in UK alcohol and tobacco industries	164
Table 8.5:	A comparison of brewing and tobacco companies	167
Table 8.6:	The concentration of ownership in the major UK alcohol and tobacco companies in 1984	169
Table 8.7:	Industry profitability	170
Table 9.1:	Average retail price of a bottle of whisky 1986/87	181
Table 9.2:	Consumption of home produced spirits (million litres of pure alcohol)	184
Table 9.3:	Rates of growth of Scotch whisky exports	184
Table 9.4:	DCL's estimated share of the home whisky market	185
Table 9.5:	Foreign ownership of distilleries 1960-1980	186
Table 9.6:	Estimated operating profits of major drinks companies (wines & spirits excluding beer, 1986)	188
Table 9.7:	Company ownership of distilleries 1978-1987	189
Table 9.8:	Estimated UK whisky market shares 1987 (by volume)	190
Table 9.9:	Scotch whisky production 1951-1986 (million litres pure alcohol)	191
Table 9.10:	Number of employees in DCL 1975-1985 (UK employees only)	192
Table 9.11:	Manpower employed in the Scotch whisky industry (1978)	193
Table 9.12:	Employment in the spirit distilling and compounding sector 1951-1985	194
Table 9.13:	Exports of Scotch whisky and Northern Irish whiskey (1946- 1986)	195
Table 9.14:	Estimated world sales of whiskies 1976	197
Table 9.15:	Major export markets for Scotch whisky (1986)	197
Table 9.16:	Taxation on Scotch whisky (per 75 cl. bottle)	198
Table 9.17:	Duty charged per centilitre of pure alcohol for five different types of drink	199

Table 9.18:   Major purchases by the Scotch whisky industry   201
              1979 (as a % of each industry's total domestic
              output and £mn)
Table 9.19:   Tax revenues from spirit expenditure   201
Table 10.1:   An information framework   206
Table 10.2:   UK employment   209
Table 10.3:   Employment in retailing   212
Table 10.4:   Total requirements per 1,000 units of final   214
              industrial output in terms of gross output
Table 10.5:   Number of operatives and administrative,   217
              clerical and technical employees, UK
Table 10.6:   Male/female employment in tobacco and   218
              alcohol industries, GB
Table 10.7:   Wages and salaries of operatives and   220
              administrative technical and clerical staff by
              industry, UK
Table 10.8:   Regional distribution of employment 1984, GB   221
Table 10.9:   Location of principal tobacco manufacturing   223
              plants, 1988

Figure 10.1:   Prevention policies and unemployment   207

List of contributors

Rob Baggott*	Lecturer in Politics, Leicester Polytechnic Research Fellow, University of Hull (1983-85)
Mark Booth*	Research Fellow, University of York (1984-86)
Christine Godfrey*	Research Fellow, University of York (1983-88)
Geoff Hardman*	Statistical Assistant, University of York (half time: 1983-88)
Larry Harrison*	Research Fellow, University of York (1983-88)
Keith Hartley	Professor of Economics, University of York
Wendy Leedham*	Research Fellow, University of Hull (1986-88)
Alan Maynard	Professor of Economics, University of York
Melanie Powell	Lecturer in Economics, Leeds Polytechnic; Research Fellow, University of York (1983-86)
David Robinson	Professor of Health Studies, University of Hull
Philip Tether*	Senior Research Fellow, University of Hull (1984- 88)
Ron Weir	Lecturer in Economic and Social History, University of York

* The asterisk indicates those Addiction Research Centre Staff who were financed by the Economic and Social Research Council.

Foreword

Preventing Alcohol and Tobacco Problems

Volume 1. The Addiction Market: consumption, production and policy development

Volume 2. Manipulating Consumption: information, law and voluntary controls

The two volumes on *Preventing Alcohol and Tobacco Problems* (each published separately) are the products of the Economic and Social Research Council-funded programme of work of the Addiction Research Centre at the Universities of Hull and York during the period 1983–1988. In addition to these volumes the staff of the Centre have published another five books and over 80 articles on various social science aspects of addiction.

The Addiction Research Centre

Addiction research presents a wide range of stimulating challenges for biomedical, clinical and social scientists. The Addiction Research Centre (ARC) in Hull-York is primarily concerned with socio-economic, policy and service issues and has focused its work particularly on the analysis of the obstacles to the creation of prevention policies which identify both their costs and benefits. The majority of projects which make up the ARC's activities are concerned with alcohol and tobacco. However, researchers in the group are also working on social science aspects of drugs, both licit (pharmaceuticals) and illicit.

Funding for the staff of economists, political scientists, health and social policy analysts and others employed in the Centre, comes from a variety of public and private sources. Most funding is short-term from Research Councils, government departments such as the Department of Health and the Home Office and other bodies such as the Institute for Alcohol Studies, the Health Promotion Research Trust and the Health Education (Council) Authority. The major grant, so far, has been from the Economic and Social Research Council (ESRC) for the five year programme of work concerned with national prevention policy which is reported on in these two volumes.

In addition to the ESRC programme, the researchers in the ARC have conducted projects concerned with problem drinkers and the statutory services; volunteer alcoholism counselling; the prevention of alcohol problems at the local level; the identification of high alcohol using patients in a District Hospital and the evaluation (cost-effectiveness) of intervention policies; the quantification of the prices, quality and volume of illicit drugs traded in the UK and the cost-effectiveness of police and Customs and Excise control policies; the analysis of European integration on the markets for alcohol and tobacco; and several aspects of the social costs of alcohol and tobacco use.

The external working relations of ARC staff are extensive and include close contact with funders and with the national bodies and professional associations concerned with addiction problems. Advice has been given by staff members to, among others, the Royal Colleges, House of Lords Select Committees, the European Economic Community and World Health Organisation. In 1986 the Hull-York group, together with the Department of Health Education at Leeds Polytechnic, was designated as a *WHO Collaborating Centre for Research and Training in the Psychosocial and Economic Aspects of Health* in recognition of our work on addictions and other health issues.

The ESRC programme

The ESRC Programme in Addiction Research was established in 1983 following the report on Research Priorities in Addiction by the Council's Exploratory Panel on Addiction. The authors of the Report believed that addiction problems are not trivial, that they are the legitimate concern of the social sciences, and that a multidisciplinary approach could reasonably be expected not only to be of interest to the social sciences but also to produce guides to policy alternatives and national strategy. After competitive tendering, the Hull-York Centre was chosen as the site for a programme concerned with 'the identification and minimisation of impediments to co-ordinated approaches to the prevention of alcohol and tobacco-related problems'. Stage I of the programme, from 1983–1986, was made up of three closely-related projects which focused on current prevention policy, the policy formation process, and industrial structures and activity.

During Stage II of the programme, 1986–1988, the insights and analyses of Stage I were used to illuminate policy choices and identify the barriers to co-ordinated national prevention policy and the factors which might mitigate them. In particular, attention was paid to the role of price regulation; the role of information, public opinion and education; and the role of legal and voluntary controls, with liquor licensing, drinking and driving, advertising and sports sponsorship as some of the specific cases in point. In addition to the policy specific work, the programme was designed to demonstrate the value of different social science disciplines being brought together to address common issues of intellectual interest and national concern.

This process has been challenging: to enable the overall multidisciplinary aim of the programme to be carried forward, while at the same time allowing the specific disciplinary skills of the staff to be brought to bear in the particular projects for which they had prime responsibilities, is not an easy task. If this has worked at all successfully it is because continuous and vigorous efforts were made to maintain a well-structured system of internal communication. In practice, this meant meeting together regularly formally and informally, exploiting each other's knowledge and skills to develop arguments and revise analyses; developing a common data base; and working closely with those on other addiction research projects and with our associates in Hull and York. The development of a research agenda and work practices across two institutions which are thirty-five miles apart has stimulated all the Hull-York researchers to ensure that communications are efficient.

Throughout the ESRC programme there have been monthly ARC meetings, alternating between Hull and York, at which the overall progress of each project has been discussed and the Centre's administrative and housekeeping issues managed. All project staff also meet together monthly and there was a full programme of seminars attended by all staff. Some of these seminars were 'closed' because the speakers reported 'off the record' to the ARC researchers about their personal involvement in core policy issues. Just as it has been vital to meet together regularly to discuss ARC organisation and project progress, it was also important for the establishment of the Centre's coherence and liveliness for all members to produce regular working papers for their colleagues' information and comments, as well as external publications (see the ARC Bibliography at the end of this volume.)

The data which were accumulated in connection with the wide range of Hull-York addiction research are stored in the ARC Data Bank. The main runs deal with alcohol and tobacco use since 1960 and related issues such as price, taxation, production, employment, distribution, advertising, offences, mortality, morbidity, public opinion and accidents. These and other data have already formed the basis of sixteen of the regular series of Data Notes published in the *British Journal of Addiction* (1986–1988).

The rationale of the overall programme of work was that it would have clear implications for policy and the prevention of problems associated with the consumption of addictive substances and clear implications also for the social sciences. The pay-offs for policy and prevention will be in terms of a better understanding of *de facto* national prevention policy, the policy formation process, relevant industrial structures and activities and the construction of strategies for the prevention of alcohol and tobacco-related problems. The pay-offs for the social sciences will be in terms of the range of detailed case studies in the politics, administration and economics of prevention, health, organizations, policy and industry. Both the policy insight and the methodological challenges form a stimulating and extensive agenda for future social science work on addictive substances.

David Robinson, Institute for Health Studies, University of Hull

Alan Maynard, Centre for Health Economics, University of York

Co-Directors ESRC Addiction Research Centre (1983–1988)

January 1989

Acknowledgements

We would like to express our thanks to the very many people who have made it possible for us to complete what many felt, at the beginning, was a very ambitious programme. That it has been completed at all satisfactorily is due to:

the ESRC programme staff,
Rob Baggott (1983–1986)
Roy Boakes (1983–1984)
Mark Booth (1985–1987)
Christine Godfrey (1983–1988)
Geoffrey Hardman (1984–1988) part-time
Larry Harrison (1983–1988)
Wendy Leedham (1986–1988) part-time
Melanie Powell (1987–1988) part-time
Philip Tether (1985–1988)

the Associates of the ARC who gave us so much sound advice,
Andy Alaszewski
Keith Hartley
Edward Page
Gilbert Smith
Albert Weale
Ron Weir

our ESRC Advisors who were always so helpful and encouraging,
Nicholas Deakin
Griffith Edwards
Julian Le Grand
Gerry Stimson

and the support staff in Hull and York who provided so much more than just secretarial expertise
Sarah Boocock (1987–1988)
Sally Cuthbert (1986–1988)
Valerie Hurst (1983–1987)
Judith Landers (1983–1986)

Special thanks are also due to Lorna Foster for copy-editing the volume, to Vanessa Windass for preparing the manuscript, and to the far-too-many-to-mention individual members of government departments, trade associations, service organisations, and others, who so generously gave us their time and interest in our attempts to understand the policy process in relation to the prevention of alcohol and tobacco problems.

Editors' introduction

ALAN MAYNARD AND PHILIP TETHER

This book, the first of two volumes, of closely linked, independent analyses of the alcohol and tobacco markets offers a substantive analysis of the factors which influence consumption, both economic and political, and the consequences of alterations in consumption patterns. During the last quarter of a century alcohol consumption has waxed whilst tobacco consumption has waned. The influence of economic and political variables on these consumption trends is not insubstantial. The tobacco industry has lost sales because the health message has been sold effectively despite adverse economic influences such as reduced real prices and enhanced purchasing power that might have been expected to increase sales. The alcohol industry has gained sales due to the increased purchasing power of consumers and the reduced real prices of wine and spirit products.

The economic self interest of both sets of producers is strong and the machinery of government is poorly designed to evaluate the health-wealth costs and benefits involved. Decision making in government departments is fragmented and compartmentalised and these characteristics are exploited by producer lobbies anxious to avoid loss of profits.

Policy formation is often difficult because of narrow objective setting, inadequate comprehension of the complexities of the market. The impediments to prevention policies in the markets for alcohol and tobacco are analysed with care and in detail in this volume.

Any discussion of consumption policy must start with an examination of consumption trends and the taxation choices of governments which thereby manipulate the tax price of alcohol and tobacco products. In Chapter 1, Geoff Hardman and Alan Maynard present an extensive array of consumption and tobacco data.

These data show that there are no 'simple facts'. For example, the consumption trends for alcohol and tobacco over the period since 1960 depend on whether value or volume series are used to measure the change in the use of these products. Expenditure on alcoholic drinks increased by 122 per cent in real terms over the period 1960–1987 (Table 1.1) but alcohol consumption by volume, measured in terms of litres of alcohol per capita for the population aged 15 years and over grew by 63 per cent (Table 1.5).

The data in this chapter demonstrate that the markets for alcohol and tobacco have altered radically over recent decades; for example, over 90 per cent of the UK population drink alcohol but between 1972 and 1986 the number of males who smoked fell from 52 per cent to 35 per cent of the population and the number of females smokers fell also, from 41 to 31 per cent (Table 1.7). In addition the market shares of particular alcohol products has changed too, with the brewers losing out to the distillers and vintners.

The relationship between these changes in the size and composition of the markets for alcohol products and tobacco and prices, income and taxation is explored descriptively in Chapter 1. It is shown that the real price of beer has increased whilst that of tobacco, wine and spirits has declined. The effects of changes in purchasing power on access to these commodities is explored for various working groups.

The apparently capricious use of taxation policies is described and it is shown that whilst the flow of tax revenue is considerable from both products, their relative importance has declined as a percentage of Central Government current account receipts (Table 1.12).

The description of consumption trends and their association with trends in prices, purchasing power and taxation gives an essential factual background but offers no insights into the relationships between these variables. The complexities of modelling demand are explored by Christine Godfrey in Chapter 2 where she demonstrates the scope for error and biased estimates of price, income and other elasticities and presents a review of past studies as well as some new estimates.

This analysis demonstrates that elasticities vary according to whether expenditure or volume measures of consumption are used, according to the time period from which data are derived, and according to the specification of the model. An array of estimates are presented. These show that the impact of price (in terms of nominal own price or relative own price) on wine and spirits consumption is significant but wide-ranging and that the estimates

2

of the income elasticities vary depending on which consumption series (expenditure or volume) is used.

As in Chapter 1 it is shown that the simplistic use of statistics may lead to naive policy conclusions and that economic analysis can illuminate relationships in a way which facilitates informed policy formation.

Any process of policy formation begs the definition of the objectives of such activity. The goals of government policy are many and various and change over time (for instance the voting consequences of tax policy will be of more importance just before elections rather than just after them). In Chapter 3 Christine Godfrey and Larry Harrison examine the objectives of government policy and seek to illuminate their interaction. They start by analysing why governments might seek to reduce the use of particular products. One possible reason for government intervention is that the users of addictive substances may impose costs on innocent third parties. Any discussion of such 'external costs' as a rationale for public policy begs the question of the definition of the externality and has to confront the problem of paternalism: if I wish to drink myself to death by over-use of alcohol, why should my freedom to do so be constrained by others?

Obviously government policy formation will also be affected by the needs for tax revenue, by the effects of tax policy on industry, trade and employment and on the distribution of the tax burden between the rich and the poor. However, these goals are often ignored, particularly by the health lobbyists with their narrow perspective.

The selection and ranking of policy objectives is a continuous state of flux with governments pursuing a mixture of policies. In particular, taxation policies vary over time according to the nature of succeeding Governments and the priorities of the moment. Godfrey and Harrison address the nature and effects of tax policies: revalorisation, increasing real rates of taxation and benchmark policies. The impact of these policies and the effects of possible European Community harmonisation policies are analysed and the (sometimes large) impact on taxes demonstrated.

The authors of Chapter 3 demonstrate that taxation is a potent mechanism influencing the use of alcohol and tobacco. However as Larry Harrison and Philip Tether show in Chapter 4, the policy process viewed from the perspective of bureaucratic politics is dominated by administrators. Advice on taxation issues in the alcohol and tobacco areas is virtually the preserve of a handful of officials in Customs and Excise and the Treasury, with mandarins elsewhere in Whitehall village having relatively little effect on policy choices. Political choice is reduced to a technical choice, with power resting in the hands of a few administrators in one very small part of the government machine. These administrators favour flexibility of choice and

3

the avoidance of rules so that the Chancellor's discretion in policy choice is as wide as possible.

This monopolisation of advice by a few officials leads to 'organisational parochialism'. If this process is to be widened to increase the flow of health information associated with the use of alcohol and tobacco, either new specialist advice has to be inserted into the existing system or the actors in the present system need to be convinced of the merits of a more catholic discussion which trades off systematically the wealth interests of producers against the health interests of users and those affected by the use of alcohol and tobacco.

The processes and outcomes of policy formation in the period since 1974 is examined by Wendy Leedham and Christine Godfrey in Chapter 5. The authors discuss the role of the health and trade lobbies and demonstrate how their interactions have become increasingly sophisticated and active; a reflection of this is the increasing number of Parliamentary questions asked about alcohol and tobacco interests. The substantial interest of Parliamentarians in this subject is paralleled by increased monitoring of public opinion. The influence of public attitudes on drink-driving and other issues has become increasingly apparent and influential in the policy process.

The authors review budgetary policy since 1974 and demonstrate the reluctance of Chancellors, both Conservative and Labour, to raise alcohol and tobacco taxes in pre-election years. Furthermore it is apparent from an analysis of Messrs Healey, Howe and Lawson's pronouncements that their major interest was and is the scope to manipulate tax rates and tax revenue for macro-economic purposes and not health issues. Thus whilst Parliament and public opinion appear to have become more concerned recently with health issues, the impact of these views on tax policy has been limited.

Some other lessons from the tax policy choices in the period 1974–1988 are also apparent. Labour Governments appear to be more concerned with the distributional effects of raising alcohol and tobacco prices, that is, protecting the poor. The Conservatives have been influenced by employment issues such as those arising from the protection of the Scotch whisky industry. Overall, however, the message is similar to that in Chapter 4: tax policy formation is an isolated process dominated by a few administrators in two powerful Government departments who have not been influenced greatly by the advocacy of the health lobbies.

The mechanisms of the political system and the actors involved in the health/producer debate and the addiction market are further investigated by Rob Baggott in Chapter 6. He examines the role of politicians, including the parliamentary membership, some 100 MPs, associated with the health lobby Action on Smoking and Health (ASH) and the links between individual MPs on both sides of the House and producer interests.

The nature of these party political and lobby influences on policy involve 'trading' by all the actors involved. This process can be confrontational. The health lobbies, due to inefficiencies in the presentation of their arguments, can easily create an adverse image, laying themselves open to the accusation that they are dictating lifestyles and curtailing individual freedom. The producer lobbies can and do respond with rhetoric about the economic consequences of prevention policies. But as Rob Baggott points out, the politics of confrontation may be inappropriate and unhelpful for the alcohol industry. Prevention is not always a zero sum game.

The future prosperity of the alcohol and tobacco industries is dependent on the negotiations its representatives and managers conduct with many Whitehall Departments. There are sixteen departments involved in the formulation of alcohol policies and Philip Tether and Larry Harrison demonstrate in Chapter 7 that they operate in virtual ignorance of each others' interests and activities and concentrate on serving their 'clients'. For instance the Ministry of Agriculture, Fisheries and Food, the Department of Trade and Industry and the Department of Employment all defend producer interests vigorously, with whom they have close and exclusive relationships.

Such Departmental-client relationships typify much of government activity but in the alcohol and tobacco fields they create impediments to the development of a coordinated prevention policy. The obstacles to such a policy are entrenched in the functionally differentiated departmental structure which may serve individual producers and departmental needs well, but which frustrate the enhancement of public health.

In Chapter 8, Mark Booth, Keith Hartley and Melanie Powell provide a detailed analysis of the structure, conduct and performance of the alcohol and tobacco industries, and indicate some of the problems associated with health promotion policies. Throughout both industries, the concentration of ownership is considerable. The largest five brewers controlled over 50 per cent of the market in both 1963 and 1985, and the top five tobacco firms controlled over 99 per cent of the market in both 1963 and 1985. The profitability of tobacco companies is high with the companies in both industries integrating vertically and horizontally as part of large multinational companies.

This chapter shows quite clearly that some of the characteristics of both industries are changing as a result of mergers and diversification, whilst others, such as profitability, are being maintained. It also shows that the economic power of these industries is considerable and international. Control policies put at risk considerable wealth and thus the industries' managers have to act vigorously to defend their shareholders interests. Ultimately, responses by producers to prevention policies depend on the effects on profits. If profits from the sales of alcohol and tobacco decline, investment and jobs will be switched over time to other (more profitable) product areas. However, concentration of economic and political power may sustain the profitability of these industries for a considerable period to come.

The particular challenges faced by the Scotch whisky industry in a decade in which prevention policies may develop rapidly is examined in Chapter 9 by Mark Booth and Ron Weir. This case study of one alcohol industry illustrates many of the problems of prevention policy. Whisky matures over a long period and consequently controls which affect consumption in the 1990s may result in producers being over-stocked for many years: this is not a new problem as consumption fell by 48 per cent between 1978 and 1983.

Reduced whisky consumption would also affect employment, much of it in rural Scotland, and lead to the concentration of production facilities. However these effects would be influenced by the relationships between domestic use and overseas sales. The latter might be influenced by domestic successes or failures, the 'shop window effect', and by reduced economies which would increase world whisky prices and hence reduce sales overseas.

Booth and Weir demonstrate that many of the propositions of the producers and health lobbyists are difficult to substantiate due to lack of clarity in their formulation and the absence of relevant information. Reducing the consumption of whisky in the UK would have significant effects on the industry and the economy and the health gains are not easy to identify and value.

Similar problems of identification and quantification arise in trying to determine the employment associated with the production and sale of alcohol and tobacco. The final chapter analyses the consequences of consumption changes for employment in the addiction market. The picture is complex, with direct employment associated with production being far less than indirect employment arising from the distribution and sales of alcohol and tobacco. As Christine Godfrey and Keith Hartley emphasise in Chapter 10 the empirical basis for the multiplier assumptions (i.e. is indirect employment seven times or eight times greater than direct employment as the industries claim?) is contentious. In terms of full-time equivalents, the authors argue that the maximum indirect employment effects are over 117,000 and 20,700 respectively in the markets for alcohol and tobacco.

An analysis of job losses in brewing and tobacco indicates that past losses have been amongst operatives, women in the tobacco industry and in plants located in high unemployment areas. In future potential losers may be highly paid workers in capital intensive plants where both owners and workers have much to lose from prevention policies. Consequently it is likely that their resistance will be intense.

In this first volume of work produced by the researchers in the joint Hull-York Addiction Research Centre, the behaviour and perspectives of competing groups, users, producers and politicians, are analysed and shown to be both highly complex and interdependent. The factors which influence the use of alcohol and tobacco, both political and economic, interact with the supply side of the market. One person's demand for these products is another person's profit and the health-wealth trade-offs are significant although often implicit in all these markets. These complex relationships make the formulation of consumption policy in the addiction market difficult for governments anxious to maintain their power by manipulating policy to their advantage, and are far removed from the simplistic generalisations of the health lobbies. Indeed the authors of each chapter in this volume demonstrate how much of the contemporary debate about alcohol and tobacco policies is based on myths and rhetoric rather than on scientific analysis and conclusions produced by careful research.

1 Consumption and taxation trends

GEOFF HARDMAN AND ALAN MAYNARD

The purpose of this chapter is to review the trends in the consumption and taxation of alcohol and tobacco over the period from 1960 to 1987. Many of the implications arising from these trends, for instance the causes of variations in consumption patterns over time, will be analysed in detail in subsequent chapters. In this chapter the time trends in consumption, prices, income and taxation will be set out and some general patterns illuminated.

CONSUMPTION TRENDS

Data on the consumption of alcohol and tobacco products have been recorded in the UK for the past two hundred years in a variety of forms and commentators have related trends in these data to specific events and social changes. During the last twenty years there has been a growing interest in issues associated with the use of alcohol and tobacco which has created a demand for more detailed data on consumption patterns. The effect of the use of alcohol and tobacco products on health, work, crime, and accidents, are areas of considerable policy interest, as is the importance in the UK economy of the alcohol and tobacco industries and the revenue received from taxation.

The actual data required to support this interest are not always available and consequently public debates are often ill-informed (McDonnell and Maynard, 1985). The need to collect data is a point taken up all too slowly by those in positions to record detailed information on particular issues, and the impetus to increase the stock of knowledge in the field of alcohol and tobacco use is changing very slowly.

There are several reasons for choosing the 1960 starting date in this chapter. Prior to 1960 data series are either not available in any detail or do not exist. The early 1960s was also a period of much standardisation of official statistics, a process which introduced a measure of consistency into the recording of data and increasing the legitimacy of time series analysis.

MEASURES OF CONSUMPTION

Consumption can be quantified by measures of volume or expenditure. Volume consumption enumerates the physical quantity of a good sold, whilst consumer expenditure measures the monetary value of such goods. Neither type of measure exactly represents consumption as neither accounts for stockpiling of goods. However, they may be said to approximate consumption, particularly when trends over time are being considered, rather than using specific figures.

A problem of consistency exists with both the volume and expenditure measures which are used in time series analysis. The product being considered does not necessarily remain the same over any length of time. The most popular brand of cigarette in 1960 may not have much relevance in 1987 when new brands have been introduced and tastes have changed. Similarly, the fashion for different alcoholic drinks changes frequently and the introduction of foreign lagers over the last twenty years has appreciably affected the traditional beer trade.

Consumer expenditure

Consumer expenditure is a function of the volume of a good sold and a unit price of that good. Over time monetary value varies and so in order to compare expenditure figures any time series must be controlled (i.e. deflated by the retail price index) for such changes. In Table 1.1 levels of total consumer expenditure of alcohol and tobacco are presented at constant 1980 prices.

Real expenditure in alcohol expenditure increased 123 per cent between 1960 and 1987, rising steadily until 1979, falling until 1982, and then rising again until 1987, when it regained its 1979 level. The trends for individual

9

Table 1.1
Consumer expenditure on alcoholic drinks and tobacco at constant 1980 prices: £ million

Year	Alcoholic Drink	Beer	Spirits	Wine, Cider & Perry	Tobacco
1960	4750	3409		1479	5051
1961	5103	3601		1640	5126
1962	5210	3672		1679	4936
1963	5388	3705	1192	632	5095
1964	5738	3876	1287	712	5026
1965	5686	3907	1236	695	4842
1966	5911	4032	1282	749	4997
1967	6154	4165	1304	841	5023
1968	6483	4301	1396	933	5003
1969	6609	4558	1330	913	4943
1970	7073	4718	1559	956	4934
1971	7544	4941	1654	1105	4759
1972	8122	5098	1883	1258	5017
1973	9211	5394	2334	1522	5309
1974	9435	5396	2495	1564	5247
1975	9350	5567	2378	1459	4995
1976	9448	5623	2325	1554	4821
1977	9487	5467	2428	1618	4602
1978	9930	5548	2616	1766	4982
1979	10382	5588	2890	1904	4960
1980	9954	5320	2720	1914	4822
1981	9612	5000	2561	2051	4470
1982	9370	4825	2427	2118	4128
1983	9730	4914	2494	2322	4083
1984	9983	4943	2525	2515	3944
1985	10224	4934	2658	2632	3837
1986	10297	4935	2646	2716	3731
1987	10574	4987	2716	2871	3704

Source: Central Statistical Office – National Income and Expenditure Accounts.

types of alcoholic drink over this same period of time do not follow the combined trend effect. Real expenditure on beer rose by 46 per cent, peaking in 1976, having increased 65 per cent from its 1960 level. It then fell 12 per cent by 1983 and has stayed at a constant level since then. Real expenditure on spirits has increased by 128 per cent since 1963, rising steadily until 1974 and then levelling off. It rose again in the late 1970s, peaking in 1979 and then decreasing until 1984. In the last few years it has increased again. Real expenditure on wines, cider and perry has shown a very different trend over the same period. Expenditure rose by 354 per cent between 1963 and 1987 and, apart from a slight decrease in 1975, has shown a continuous and steady increase.

In contrast to consumer expenditure on alcohol, real expenditure on tobacco has decreased since 1960. Between 1960 and 1987 real tobacco expenditure decreased by 27 per cent with almost all of this decreasing occurring since 1980. Between 1960 and 1980 there was no appreciable change in expenditure on tobacco.

Relative expenditure

To show the differences between the various alcohol products the expenditure figures are best presented in relative terms. Table 1.2 shows product shares of the total alcoholic drink market.

In 1960, expenditure on beer accounted for 58.8 per cent of all expenditure on alcohol, expenditure on spirits 29.6 per cent, and expenditure on wines, cider and perry 11.5 per cent. Between 1960 and 1987 expenditure on beer fell to 52.8 per cent of all expenditure on alcohol, expenditure on spirits fell to 24.3 per cent, whereas expenditure on wines, cider and perry rose to 22.9 per cent of the total. The percentage of the market from beer sales held constant from 1960 to 1972 but then dropped suddenly in the mid 1970s before picking up again, though with an underlying trend downwards. The market share (as a percentage of expenditure) of spirits shows a steadily declining market share from 1960 to 1971, a sudden increase in 1973 followed by a further steady decline. Closer examination of the shares of beer and spirits in the alcohol market suggests a degree of product switching between the two. As the share of beer varies up or down, the share of spirits varies conversely. Both beer and spirits lost market share to wines, cider and perry. Apart from a levelling out between 1975 and 1980, the market share of wines, cider and perry has increased steadily over the period taking equally from beer and spirits.

As well as considering variations between disaggregations of alcohol and tobacco expenditure, consideration of expenditure on alcohol and tobacco relative to other commodities is relevant to a fuller understanding of the consumption patterns of these products. Table 1.3 shows how the proportions of alcohol and tobacco in total consumer expenditure have changed over the period.

The share of expenditure on alcohol in total consumer expenditure rose from 5.7 per cent in 1960 to 6.8 per cent in 1987, increasing steadily until 1976, when it was 7.7 per cent, and decreasing slightly from 1977 to 1987. The share of tobacco expenditure in total expenditure has steadily declined from 6.7 per cent in 1960 to 3.0 per cent in 1987.

11

Table 1.2

Product shares in the alcohol industry as percentages of the total alcoholic drink market

Year	Beer	Spirits	Wines, Cider & Perry
1960	58.8	29.6	11.5
1961	58.0	30.4	11.5
1962	59.2	30.1	10.8
1963	58.2	28.8	13.0
1964	57.0	29.3	13.7
1965	58.8	28.0	13.1
1966	58.5	27.9	13.7
1967	58.7	27.1	14.2
1968	57.1	27.8	15.2
1969	59.2	25.6	15.2
1970	58.9	26.6	14.5
1971	58.9	25.8	15.3
1972	57.1	26.7	16.2
1973	52.8	29.3	17.9
1974	52.9	28.7	18.4
1975	55.2	27.6	17.2
1976	57.0	25.9	17.1
1977	57.0	26.2	16.8
1978	56.0	26.5	17.4
1979	54.7	27.4	17.9
1980	55.8	26.5	17.8
1981	55.9	25.2	18.8
1982	56.4	24.2	19.5
1983	57.2	23.3	19.6
1984	54.0	23.9	22.1
1985	53.3	24.5	22.2
1986	53.7	24.2	22.1
1987	52.8	24.3	22.9

Source: Central Statistical Office – National Income and Expenditure Accounts.

Volume consumption

The source of volume data on alcohol and tobacco products is principally HM Customs and Excise and the information refers to the quantities of products released from bond. Table 1.4 shows the volume measures of beer, spirits, wines, and cider in the period from 1960 to 1987.

The consumption of beer increased by 39 per cent, that of spirits by 153 per cent, that of wine by 462 per cent, and that of cider by 241 per cent over

Table 1.3

Expenditure on alcoholic drinks and tobacco as a percentage of total consumer expenditure

Year	Alcoholic drink	Tobacco
1960	5.7	6.7
1961	6.0	6.8
1962	6.1	6.6
1963	6.1	6.4
1964	6.5	6.3
1965	6.5	6.2
1966	6.7	6.2
1967	6.8	5.9
1968	6.8	5.7
1969	6.9	5.8
1970	7.2	5.4
1971	7.3	4.8
1972	7.2	4.5
1973	7.5	4.2
1974	7.4	4.2
1975	7.5	4.2
1976	7.7	4.1
1977	7.7	4.2
1978	7.5	3.9
1979	7.6	3.6
1980	7.5	3.6
1981	7.6	3.6
1982	7.4	3.6
1983	7.5	3.4
1984	7.4	3.4
1985	7.4	3.3
1986	7.0	3.2
1987	6.8	3.0

Source: Central Statistical Office—National Income and Expenditure Accounts.

the period. The trend in beer consumption shows a steady increase until 1979, followed by an equally steady decrease up to 1987. The overall trend in spirits consumption shows a peak in 1979 as the beer trend does. However, prior to 1979 spirits sales show very little change until 1970 and then double from 1970 to 1979. From 1979 the sales of spirits decrease though only slightly. Apart from a period of no change in the mid 1970s the sales of wine have increased steadily with a gradual acceleration of the trend over the period. Cider sales have also increased steadily though the figures show this trend

13

Table 1.4

Consumption of alcoholic drink: quantities released for home consumption—million litres

Year	Beer	Spirits[a]	Wines	Cider[b]
1960	4460.3	38.7	121.7	85.9
1961	4656.8	40.9	129.2	91.4
1962	4676.5	41.2	133.1	82.7
1963	4696.1	44.0	147.9	83.2
1964	4912.3	47.7	169.1	86.8
1965	4971.2	45.5	161.5	90.5
1966	5049.8	46.2	171.9	100.9
1967	5148.1	46.5	189.3	113.6
1968	5246.3	48.3	211.2	116.8
1969	5462.5	45.5	204.1	130.5
1970	5639.3	52.1	208.4	142.7
1971	5855.4	55.2	245.0	143.2
1972	5993.0	63.0	281.5	144.1
1973	6268.1	78.6	356.3	156.4
1974	6405.6	86.4	376.5	158.2
1975	6562.8	82.3	352.4	184.1
1976	6654.0	92.5	367.0	215.9
1977	6589.2	79.1	356.0	203.7
1978	6780.0	95.8	420.1	207.3
1979	6824.4	105.5	454.3	214.1
1980	6549.6	99.6	453.7	211.4
1981	6231.6	94.6	486.7	229.6
1982	6140.4	89.2	490.8	272.3
1983	6223.2	91.7	535.8	303.2
1984	6208.0	91.2	589.0	303.2
1985	6150.1	97.4	618.1	292.3
1986	6120.6	96.8	643.0	298.2
1987	6197.4	98.1	684.0	293.2

a. Million litres of pure alcohol. Since 1st January 1980, H.M. Customs and Excise have published volume data in terms of pure alcohol. No average strength figures are published and so it is not strictly possible to convert litres of pure alcohol into bulk litres.

b. Until 6th September 1976 there was no excise duty on cider. Consequently, there are no official statistics on production or consumption. The figures above are for sales of National Association members.

Source: Monthly Digest of Statistics, The Brewers Society: UK. Statistical Handbook.

levelling off since 1983. As with the expenditure series, Table 1.4 shows the increased market share of wines and cider over beer and spirits.

Relative comparisons in volume series for alcohol are often standardised for alcoholic content. In Table 1.5, consumption is shown in terms of pure alcohol per head of population aged 15 and over. It can be seen that the total per capita intake of alcohol increased from 6.0 to 10.2 litres between 1960 and 1979 and, although it then started dropping, it has been increasing again in the last few years.

In 1960, 73.7 per cent of pure alcohol consumed was from beer, 16.8 per cent from spirits, 6.7 per cent from wines, and 2.8 per cent from cider, with a total of 6.0 litres of pure alcohol per head of population aged 15 and over. By 1987 the total volume of alcohol consumed had increased by 63 per cent to 9.8 litres of pure alcohol per head of population aged 15 and over. Of this total, 55.0 per cent was from beer, 21.4 per cent from spirits, 18.3 per cent from wines, and 5.2 per cent from cider.

The volume series for tobacco consumption can be expressed in terms of number and weight. However, due to considerable changes in the tobacco market over the past twenty years both types of series have the problem of comparability of data. The switch from plain to filter cigarettes followed by the move to low tar brands has meant significant changes in the amount of tobacco per average cigarette. Table 1.6 shows the figures for sales of cigarettes by weight and by number.

Both the series shows a general fall in consumption from 1960 to 1987, 14.3 per cent in terms of number of cigarettes, and 26.8 per cent in terms of weight of tobacco used. The variation between these figures reflects the changes in taste over the time period considered. The trends in the consumption patterns shown by the two series are also markedly different. The data on sales of cigarettes by number show an increase of 24 per cent from 1960 to 1973 followed by a decrease of 31 per cent from 1973 to 1987. Sales by weight data show a steady decline over the whole period with slight increases around 1973 and 1978.

The consumption of other tobacco products over time by weight is also shown in Table 1.6. Whereas the overall picture is one of a steady decline in sales from 1960 to 1987, sales of tobacco as cigars and cigarillos increased by 386 per cent from 1960 to 1975 and by 286 per cent overall. The sales of pipe tobacco decreased by 68 per cent in the period and sales of hand rolling tobacco decreased by 32 per cent.

Between 1975 and 1987 tobacco consumption shows a dramatic decrease whichever measure is used. The data on consumption patterns of smokers show a more gradual decrease. Table 1.7 presents the biannual data (taken from the General Household Survey) of the consumption trends of smokers broken down by age and sex.

15

Table 1.5

Consumption per capita of pure alcohol[a] (in litres per head of population aged 15 and over)—calendar year data

Year	Beer	Spirits	Wine	Cider	Total
1960	4.4	1.0	0.4	0.17	6.0
1961	4.6	1.0	0.4	0.18	6.2
1962	4.6	1.0	0.4	0.16	6.2
1963	4.6	1.1	0.4	0.16	6.3
1964	4.8	1.2	0.5	0.17	6.7
1965	4.8	1.1	0.5	0.17	6.6
1966	4.8	1.1	0.5	0.19	6.6
1967	4.9	1.1	0.5	0.22	6.7
1968	5.0	1.2	0.6	0.22	7.0
1969	5.2	1.1	0.6	0.25	7.1
1970	5.4	1.2	0.6	0.27	7.5
1971	5.6	1.3	0.7	0.27	7.9
1972	5.7	1.5	0.8	0.27	8.3
1973	5.9	1.8	1.0	0.29	9.0
1974	6.0	2.0	1.1	0.3.	9.4
1975	6.1	1.9	1.0	0.34	9.3
1976	6.1	2.1	1.0	0.40	9.6
1977	6.0	1.8	1.0	0.37	9.2
1978	6.2	2.2	1.1	0.38	9.9
1979	6.2	2.4	1.2	0.39	10.2
1980	5.9	2.2	1.2	0.38	9.7
1981	5.6	2.1	1.3	0.41	9.4
1982	5.5	2.0	1.3	0.48	9.3
1983	5.5	2.0	1.4	0.54	9.4
1984	5.5	2.0	1.6	0.53	9.6
1985	5.4	2.1	1.6	0.51	9.6
1986	5.3	2.1	1.7	0.52	9.6
1987	5.4	2.1	1.8	0.51	9.8

a. These estimates assume average alcohol content as follows:

    Beer — 4% alcohol

    Wine — 12% alcohol

    Spirits — 40% alcohol

    Cider — 8% alcohol

Sources: Annual Abstract of Statistics, The Brewers Society: UK Statistical Handbook.

Table 1.6

Consumption of tobacco products in the UK by numbers and weight

Year	Cigarettes ('000 million)	Cigarettes (Mill. Kg.)	Cigars and Cigarillos (Mill. Kg.)	Pipe tobacco (Mill. Kg.)	Hand-rolling Tobacco
1960	110.9	108.4	0.7	7.9	7.1
1961	113.4	110.3	0.7	7.4	7.3
1962	109.9	104.7	0.9	7.8	7.2
1963	115.2	107.9	1.0	7.3	7.6
1964	114.4	104.7	1.2	7.1	7.7
1965	112.0	100.1	1.3	6.6	7.3
1966	117.6	101.3	1.6	6.4	7.1
1967	119.1	100.4	1.8	6.3	7.1
1968	121.8	99.9	1.9	6.0	7.0
1969	124.9	98.2	1.9	5.9	6.8
1970	127.9	97.7	2.0	5.8	6.5
1971	122.4	92.6	2.7	6.0	5.9
1972	130.5	98.1	2.9	5.7	6.2
1973	137.4	103.8	3.3	5.6	6.1
1974	137.0	102.3	3.2	5.4	6.1
1975	132.6	96.4	3.4	5.0	6.4
1976	130.6	93.2	3.2	5.0	6.5
1977	125.9	89.7	3.0	4.9	6.5
1978	125.2	98.9	3.2	4.6	6.1
1979	124.3	98.6	3.2	4.2	5.7
1980	121.5	97.2	3.0	4.0	5.6
1981	110.3	89.4	2.9	3.8	6.2
1982	102.0	82.6	2.7	3.5	6.2
1983	101.6	83.0	2.6	3.3	5.8
1984	99.0	81.6	2.7	3.2	5.3
1985	97.8	81.1	2.6	3.0	5.0
1986	95.5	79.8	2.6	2.8	4.8
1987	95.0	79.4	2.7	2.5	4.8

Sources: Lee P.N., (ed.), (1976), Statistics of Smoking in the United Kingdom, 7th Edition (Tobacco Research Council): Tobacco Advisory Council fact sheets, 1977–1987.

Table 1.7

Average weekly cigarette consumption by current smokers by sex and age: Great Britain

Year	16–19	20–24	25–34	Age Group 35–49	50–59	60 & over	All	%
(a) Men								
1972	102	123	129	132	124	96	120	52
1974	110	132	136	138	127	100	125	51
1976	106	135	138	141	130	108	129	46
1978	98	122	134	138	137	104	127	45
1980	99	113	135	140	130	102	124	42
1982	87	114	121	137	129	109	121	38
1984	87	107	114	130	126	103	115	36
1986	86	108	110	133	120	103	115	35
(b) Women								
1972	76	91	97	94	87	60	87	41
1974	86	99	108	104	91	68	94	41
1976	89	110	109	112	103	75	101	38
1978	90	101	113	109	101	79	101	37
1980	84	102	111	115	105	73	102	37
1982	76	100	109	108	101	77	98	33
1984	80	91	105	107	98	80	96	32
1986	77	85	101	112	99	84	97	31

Source: Cigarette Smoking 1972 to 1986, OPCS Monitor. Reference SS 88/1

The trends in this table suggest that the decrease in overall tobacco consumption is caused by people giving up smoking entirely. The percentage of smokers in the population has decreased for both sexes, whereas the average number of cigarettes smoked by smokers has decreased only slightly for men and increased for women. When the smoking population is broken down by age as well as sex, it can be seen that older men have also increased their cigarette consumption. The age breakdown for women shows that although all age groups have increased their consumption, older women have increased more than young women. However, the figures show that, irrespective of sex or age, the consumption of tobacco by smokers has been falling since the late 1970s.

CONSUMPTION, PRICE AND INCOME TRENDS

The economic factors which influence the consumption patterns of alcohol and tobacco products are analysed in Chapter 2, but it can be seen from trends over time that variations in the prices of products are intrinsically linked to consumption trends. Variation over time in the price of a product is the major reason for differences between the expenditure and the volume consumption series and price series are therefore valuable in themselves. However, as with expenditure and volume consumption series, there is the problem of changes in the products over time, making it difficult to price a typical item.

One way of overcoming this problem is to consider prices over a range of goods and weight them by the expenditure shares of the individual items. This is the methodology used for constructing the Retail Price Index (RPI). Unfortunately the characteristics of the index are not published in great detail and for alcohol the only two indices available are for beer and for spirits, wines and other alcoholic drinks combined. The indices presented in Table 1.8 are calculated by comparing current expenditure series with constant priced expenditure series issued by the Central Statistical Office, the source of official statistics used for expenditure series. The figures have been rebased for 1963=100 to facilitate price comparison over the period, and are presented here relative to the 'all items' price index, (i.e. 'all items' held constant (=100) over time).

Since 1963 the cost of living as measured by the imputed price index has increased about seven fold (708 per cent). By controlling for this increase in 'all items', relative price indices are created for specific products.

Relative to 'all items' prices, the price of beer has increased 35 per cent, the price of spirits has decreased 26 per cent, and the price of wines, cider and perry has decreased 22 per cent, over the period 1963 to 1987. Up until 1980 beer prices kept pace with the 'all items' trend but since then have increased significantly. The relative price for spirits decreased steadily until 1980 when it levelled out and has, since 1980, shown a slight increase. Wine and cider prices have shown a steady decrease over the whole period relative to 'all items'.

From the early 1960s until 1974, the price of tobacco decreased relative to 'all items', picking up a little in the mid 1970s, decreasing again until 1979. Since 1979 it has increased steadily, though not until 1983 did the price of tobacco return to its 1963 level relative to 'all items'.

Apart from looking at price variations of products relative to 'all items', price series may be controlled for changes in income over time. Just as an expenditure series is better controlled for changes in monetary value in order to consider real changes, so presenting prices relative to income provides a measure of purchasing power to a price series. If people spend more on

Table 1.8

Commodity price indices relative to 'all items'—1963 = 100

Year	Beer	Spirits	Wines & Cider	Tobacco
1963	100.0	100.0	100.0	100.1
1964	101.9	102.8	102.2	102.2
1965	107.3	105.2	102.9	107.4
1966	107.7	105.2	103.2	105.5
1967	109.2	104.7	100.0	102.8
1968	105.4	102.9	98.8	102.8
1969	106.2	102.3	103.8	105.8
1970	109.2	97.1	101.3	101.7
1971	108.1	92.4	96.1	95.5
1972	107.2	88.4	94.1	90.9
1973	101.8	85.0	93.3	85.0
1974	99.7	76.2	91.2	84.6
1975	100.7	77.1	91.6	88.1
1976	104.4	75.7	87.9	89.2
1977	105.3	73.8	83.1	95.4
1978	103.7	70.9	80.8	86.6
1979	104.6	69.1	81.6	83.5
1980	109.4	69.7	80.2	84.1
1981	117.1	71.0	79.8	93.1
1982	120.0	71.3	80.1	99.0
1983	124.2	71.7	78.7	100.3
1984	128.0	73.6	79.4	105.4
1985	133.7	74.1	79.7	109.8
1986	135.5	74.0	77.6	116.2
1987	134.6	73.7	77.5	115.5

Source: Central Statistical Office—National Income and Expenditure Accounts.

alcohol and tobacco as their income rises it is necessary to consider trends in the change of income, as well as in the real price, to understand trends in consumption. Table 1.9 shows personal disposable income (PDI) per head of population aged 15 and over, and the price indices used in Table 1.8 controlled for changes in PDI, rebased to 1963=100 for ease of comparison.

Although beer prices and tobacco prices have gone up relative to 'all items' since 1960, relative to income beer prices dropped 16 per cent and tobacco prices dropped 28 per cent over the period. However, since 1980, beer prices have risen relative to income and tobacco prices have stabilised. The index produced for 'all items' shows that prices have generally fallen quite dramatically (almost 40 per cent) over the period, relative to income.

20

Table 1.9

Purchasing power: price in relation to personal disposable income

Year	Personal disposable income p.a. (15 years & over) (£) Current Prices	Current price indices as percentages of personal disposable income 1963 = 100				
		Beer	Spirits	Wine & Cider	Tobacco	All Items
1963	522	100.0	100.0	100.0	100.0	100.0
1964	564	97.7	98.6	98.0	98.0	95.9
1965	597	102.0	99.9	97.8	102.1	95.0
1966	635	100.1	97.8	95.9	98.1	93.0
1967	659	100.4	96.2	91.9	94.5	91.9
1968	699	95.7	93.4	89.7	93.3	90.8
1969	739	96.2	92.7	94.1	95.9	90.6
1970	826	93.7	83.3	86.9	87.3	85.8
1971	911	91.4	78.1	81.2	80.7	84.5
1972	1043	84.3	69.5	74.0	71.5	78.6
1973	1199	75.4	63.0	69.1	63.0	74.1
1974	1412	73.3	56.1	67.1	62.2	73.6
1975	1723	75.1	57.5	68.4	65.7	74.6
1976	1967	78.9	57.2	66.5	67.4	75.6
1977	2205	81.6	57.1	64.4	73.9	77.5
1978	2582	74.8	51.1	58.3	63.8	72.1
1979	3040	72.7	48.0	56.7	58.1	69.5
1980	3645	73.8	47.0	54.1	56.7	67.5
1981	3900	82.3	49.9	56.1	65.4	70.3
1982	4184	85.4	50.7	57.0	70.4	71.1
1983	4456	87.4	50.5	55.4	70.6	70.4
1984	4872	86.6	49.8	53.7	71.3	67.7
1985	5257	87.5	48.5	52.2	71.8	65.4
1986	5653	85.5	46.7	48.9	73.2	63.1
1987	5925	84.0	46.0	48.4	72.1	62.4

Source: Central Statistical Office—National Income and Expenditure: Monthly Digest of Statistics.

The prices for spirits, and wines and cider have dropped more than 50 per cent relative to income over the period.

An alternative way of linking prices and income is to consider the time required to earn the price of a quantity of a good, for example, the number of minutes it takes to earn the price of twenty cigarettes or a bottle of whisky. In Table 1.10, four groups of workers are considered: male manual, male non-manual, female manual, and female non-manual.

Table 1.10a

Minutes of work[a] required to earn the price of a pint of draught beer[b]

Year	Male Manual	Male Non-manual	Female Manual	Female Non-manual
1962	12.9	7.8	21.5	14.6
1963	12.7	7.6	21.2	14.3
1964	12.8	7.8	21.4	14.6
1965	13.1	7.9	22.2	14.8
1966	12.0	7.5	20.1	14.2
1967	12.4	7.6	20.7	14.4
1968	11.4	7.1	19.4	13.5
1969	11.4	7.1	19.2	13.3
1970	11.3	7.3	19.3	13.7
1971	11.2	7.3	18.8	13.6
1972	10.5	6.8	17.4	12.5
1973	9.5	6.4	15.7	11.8
1974	9.6	6.5	15.2	11.7
1975	9.6	6.7	14.3	11.0
1976	9.6	6.6	13.7	10.4
1977	10.2	7.0	14.3	11.1
1978	9.7	6.6	13.6	10.8
1979	10.1	7.1	14.6	11.5
1980	9.9	6.7	14.1	11.0
1981	10.7	7.0	15.5	11.3
1982	10.8	7.1	15.9	11.5
1983	11.2	7.3	16.3	11.8
1984	11.3	7.3	16.4	11.7
1985	11.4	7.3	16.3	11.7
1986	11.2	7.0	16.2	11.3
1987	11.1	6.8	15.9	11.1

a. Hourly earnings are estimated average hourly earnings for April of the year in question. From 1972 onwards, estimates only relate to employees whose earnings are not affected by absence from work.

b. Beer prices are mid-year prices of a pint of draught beer in a public bar and excludes premium bitters.

Sources: Department of Employment Gazette
　　　　　UK Handbook of The Brewers Society.

Table 1.10b

Hours of work[a] required to earn the price of a bottle of whisky[b]

Year	Male Manual	Male Non-manual	Female Manual	Female Non-manual
1960	6.4	3.8	10.6	7.2
1961	6.6	4.0	10.9	7.5
1962	6.3	3.8	10.5	7.1
1963	6.0	3.6	10.0	6.8
1964	6.0	3.6	10.1	6.9
1965	6.1	3.7	10.3	6.9
1966	5.9	3.7	10.0	7.0
1967	5.8	3.6	9.7	6.8
1968	5.6	3.5	9.5	6.7
1969	5.3	3.3	8.9	6.2
1970	4.8	3.1	8.1	5.8
1971	4.3	2.7	7.1	5.1
1972	3.8	2.5	6.3	4.5
1973	3.4	2.3	5.5	4.2
1974	3.1	2.1	4.9	3.8
1975	2.9	2.0	4.3	3.3
1976	2.7	1.9	3.9	3.0
1977	2.7	1.9	3.9	3.0
1978	2.5	1.7	3.4	2.7
1979	2.3	1.6	3.4	2.7
1980	2.1	1.5	3.1	2.4
1981	2.2	1.5	3.2	2.3
1982	2.2	1.4	3.2	2.3
1983	2.1	1.4	3.0	2.2
1984	2.2	1.4	3.2	2.2
1985	2.1	1.3	3.0	2.1
1986	2.0	1.3	2.9	2.0
1987	1.9	1.2	2.8	1.9

a.   See Note a on Table 1.10a.

b.   Prices are based on the price of a bottle of whisky in April of the year in question.

Sources: Department of Employment, *Employment Gazette*
            Scotch Whisky Association.

Table 1.10c

Hours of work[a] required to earn the price of a bottle of wine

Year	Male Manual	Male Non-manual	Female Manual	Female Non-manual
1974	1.0	0.7	1.6	1.2
1975	1.1	0.8	1.7	1.3
1976	1.1	0.8	1.6	1.2
1977	1.1	0.7	1.5	1.2
1978	1.0	0.7	1.4	1.1
1979	1.0	0.7	1.5	1.2
1980	1.0	0.7	1.4	1.1
1981	1.0	0.7	1.5	1.1
1982	1.0	0.7	1.5	1.1
1983	1.0	0.6	1.4	1.0
1984	0.9	0.5	1.2	0.9
1985	0.9	0.5	1.2	0.9
1986	0.9	0.5	1.2	0.9
1987	0.9	0.6	1.3	0.9

a.   See Note a on Table 1.10a

Sources: J. Sainsbury, Augustus Barnett, Marks and Spencer, Department of Employment, *Employment Gazette*.

Table 1.10d

Minutes of work[a] required to earn the price of 20 cigarettes[b]

Year	Male Manual	Male Non-manual	Female Manual	Female Non-manual
1960	32.6	19.4	54.2	36.6
1961	30.5	18.5	50.3	34.8
1962	30.8	18.6	51.5	34.9
1963	29.6	17.7	49.3	33.2
1964	30.1	18.2	50.2	34.3
1965	31.7	19.0	53.6	35.8
1966	28.9	18.2	48.6	34.2
1967	28.3	17.4	47.2	32.8
1968	26.8	16.7	45.3	31.5
1969	28.0	17.3	47.1	32.7
1970	25.2	16.2	43.0	30.5
1971	22.5	14.5	37.6	27.2
1972	20.2	13.0	33.5	24.0
1973	19.5	13.1	32.1	24.0
1974	20.5	13.9	32.4	25.0
1975	19.9	13.9	29.8	22.9
1976	17.9	12.3	25.6	19.5
1977	20.3	14.0	28.6	22.1
1978	18.8	12.8	26.3	20.9
1979	16.7	11.6	24.0	19.0
1980	17.8	12.1	25.5	19.8
1981	19.8	13.0	28.8	21.0
1982	20.5	13.4	30.1	21.8
1983	20.0	13.0	29.2	21.1
1984	21.6	13.8	31.3	22.3
1985	21.4	13.7	30.6	21.9
1986	22.2	13.9	31.9	22.3
1987	22.3	13.7	31.8	22.2

a. See Note a on Table 1.10a.

b. Up to April 1973 the price figure used in the above table is for 20 smaller cigarettes of the popular range. Between April 1973 and April 1977 the used price is for a standard size filter cigarette and the prices used for years since April 1977 are based on king size filter cigarettes—following the most popular cigarette at the time. All prices used are as for April of the year in question.

Sources: Department of Employment, *Employment Gazette*.
        Tobacco Trade Year Book.

The trends shown for each product are similar to those shown in Table 1.9. However, by separating the population into men and women, and manual and non-manual workers, the effect of income changes over time can clearly be seen to be different for these groups. The purchasing power of women workers has increased enormously in the period. This increase in prosperity for women is one of the factors associated with the increase in cigarette consumption by the female population during a period of decrease for men.

CONSUMPTION AND TAXATION TRENDS

High levels of taxation on alcohol and tobacco are a common feature of many developed economies and are an important source of government revenue in the UK. Changes in taxation can affect significantly the price of alcohol and tobacco and such changes are an important determinant of consumption. The formulation of taxation policy, a key factor in the implementation of prevention policies, is discussed in detail in Chapters 3, 4 and 5 below. Here the objective is to describe the nature and level of taxation of alcohol and tobacco in the last two decades.

There are two types of indirect taxation levied on alcoholic beverages and tobacco: an ad valorem tax on value, such as VAT; and a specific tax on quantity, such as the excise tax set at, for instance, so much (£x) per 1,000 cigarettes. Excise tax is fixed to quantity alone and varies with strength and category. Ad valorem taxes are set as a percentage of final price and, as such, are self-adjusting as prices rise. The fixed excise element must be formally adjusted at regular intervals if a decline in real values is to be avoided.

Since 1960, the structure of alcohol and tobacco taxation has undergone a series of changes. In 1973, Value Added Tax (VAT) was introduced on a wide range of products including most alcohol and tobacco goods. VAT is fixed at the point of sale as a percentage of the retail price. At the time of introduction of VAT, the specific excise elements of tax on both alcohol and tobacco were reduced so that the proportion of tax in price remained at a similar level to when the goods were subject to excise tax only.

The introduction of VAT on alcohol and tobacco meant that the amount of tax on the goods varied both with changes in specific excise taxes and the general VAT rate.

Between 1976 and 1978 further structural changes were made to the pattern of alcohol and tobacco taxation as part of a move towards tax harmonisation within the European Community (EC). Cigarettes had been taxed by weight of unmanufactured tobacco leaf but this was replaced by a specific fixed rate per 1,000 cigarettes. Wine duties had been set as an import duty with different rates for imports from the Commonwealth and non-Commonwealth countries. From the 1st January 1976, wine duty was changed to an excise duty and levied on all wines including those produced in the UK. Three levels of duty were introduced based on alcoholic content. In 1974 the EC ruled that beer and wine must be taxed at similar rates according to strength of alcohol per volume.

In Tables 1.11a and 1.11b comparisons of duty rates over time are shown for alcohol and tobacco products.

Table 1.11a

Tobacco duty rates 1960–1988

a) 1960–1978—Tobacco leaf duty

Date of Change[a]	Basic Duty (£ per lb)
5.4.60	3.225
15.4.64	3.869
7.4.65	4.369
20.3.68	4.585
1.4.73[b]	4.305
27.3.74	5.671
16.4.75	7.704
10.5.76[c]	5.832
30.3.77	6.417
1.1.78	Abolished

Table 1.11a (cont.)

b) 1976–1988—Tobacco Product Duty

Date of Change	Cigarettes		Cigars	Hand–rolling tobacco	Other smoking tobacco and chewing
	Ad valorem %	Specific per 1000 £		(£ per Kg)[f]	
10.5.76[d]	20	0	6.10	5.29	3.42
4.4.77	22	1.41	6.71	8.43	3.76
1.1.78[e]	30	9.00	20.28	20.28	16.09
13.8.79	21	11.77	20.94	20.28	16.09
29.3.80	21	13.42	25.60	22.60	17.40
14.3.81	21	18.04	34.29	29.56	21.92
8.7.81	21	19.03	35.91	30.96	22.96
12.3.82	21	20.68	39.00	33.65	24.95
18.3.83	21	21.67	40.85	35.40	24.95
16.3.84	21	24.97	47.05	43.73	24.95
22.3.85	21	26.95	47.05	43.73	24.95
18.3.86	21	30.61	47.05	43.73	24.95
15.3.88	21	31.74	48.79	51.48	24.95

a. Only the main Budget changes in basic duty shown.

b. Tobacco liable to VAT from 1.4.73.

c. Subject to 10% increase from 16.12.76 to 3.4.77. Basic rate abated by £1.855 per lb to allow for the introduction of tobacco products duty.

d. Subject to 10% increase.

e. Increased with the abolition of tobacco leaf duty.

f. Actual duty rates which were set per lb have been converted to metric equivalents from (1.5.76 to 1.1.80).

Source: HM Customs and Excise.

Table 1.11b
Alcohol duty rates 1960–1988

Beer, Spirits and Cider Duties

Date of Change	Beer		Spirits	Cider
	per hectolitre[a] at 1030	per additional degree	per litre alcohol	per hectolitre[a]
15.4.64	4.49	0.223	4.96	–
7.4.65	5.22	0.223	5.62	–
12.4.67	5.76	0.244	6.19	–
20.3.68	–	–	6.60	–
1.4.73	4.22	0.177	5.95	–
27.3.74	5.72	0.191	6.56	–
16.4.75	8.36	0.279	8.51	–
7.4.76[b]	9.68	0.327	9.49	4.84
30.3.77	10.65	0.355	10.44	5.32
27.3.80	13.05	0.435	11.87	6.05
11.3.81	18.00	0.600	13.60	7.20
10.3.82	20.40	0.680	14.47	8.16
16.3.83	21.60	0.720	15.19	9.69
14.3.84	24.00	0.800	15.48	14.28
20.3.85	25.80	0.860	15.77	15.80
15.3.88	27.00	0.900	15.77	17.33

Wine duties

Date of Change	Wine (£ per hectolitre)		Made Wine	
	Lower	Higher	Lower	Higher
10.4.62	15.40	30.25	12.65	12.65
15.4.64	17.05	33.55	14.30	14.30
7.4.65	20.35	40.15	17.60	18.70
12.4.67	22.27	43.17	19.52	21.72
20.3.68	25.57	49.77	22.82	28.32
16.4.69	35.47	59.67	32.72	38.22
1.4.73	19.25	43.45	16.50	22.00
27.3.74	30.14	51.03	28.49	33.99
16.4.75	58.84	78.09	57.74	63.24

Table 1.11b (cont)

Wine duties (cont)

Date of Change	Wine (£ per hectolitre)			Made Wine (£ per hectolitre)		
	Lower (15)	Middle (15—18)	Higher (18—22)	Lower (10)	Middle (10—15)	Higher (15—18)
7.4.76	65.01	75.02	88.33	42.24	63.25	69.52
30.3.77	71.49	82.48	97.11	46.41	69.51	76.43
27.3.80	81.42	93.93	110.59	52.85	79.16	87.04
11.3.81	95.20	122.90	144.70	61.80	92.50	113.90
10.3.82	106.80	137.90	162.30	73.10	103.80	127.80
16.3.83	113.00	145.90	171.70	79.30	109.80	135.20

	Lower (15)	Middle (15—18)	Higher (18—22)
14.3.84	90.5	157.5	183.3
20.3.85	98.0	169.0	194.9
15.3.88	102.4	176.6	203.7

a. Duties expressed in metric terms throughout to ease comparisons.

b. All duties subjected to 10% regulator surcharge 1.1.77 to 29.3.77.

Source: H.M. Customs and Excise.

The revenue from alcohol and tobacco taxes is clearly important to governments. In Table 1.12 real tax yields (i.e. tax yields adjusted to 1980 prices) are presented along with measures designed to indicate the relative importance of alcohol and tobacco as a source of revenue.

The real tax yield for alcohol has risen by 111 per cent over the period from 1960 to 1987, remaining fairly constant as a percentage of total tax on expenditure, and decreasing slightly as a percentage of total central government receipts.

Whereas in 1960 tobacco tax yielded 114 per cent more revenue than alcohol tax, in 1987 it yielded 6 per cent less revenue than alcohol. In real terms tobacco tax revenue has fallen 7 per cent since 1960. Since 1978 the yield from tobacco tax has been consistently below that of alcohol. The decline in tobacco tax is reflected more dramatically when considering it as a percentage of total tax on expenditure. In 1960 tobacco tax yielded over a quarter of all expenditure taxes and more than 10 per cent of all central

Table 1.12

Revenue from alcoholic drink and tobacco

Year	Real Tax Yields[a] (£m 1980 prices)		Alcohol Tax as % of total tax on expenditure	Tobacco Tax as % of total tax on expenditure	Alcohol Tax as % of total Central Govt. current A/C receipts	Tobacco Tax as % of total Central Govt. current A/C receipts
	Alcohol Tax	Tobacco Tax				
1960	1962	4208	13.4	28.7	5.6	11.9
1961	2102	4289	13.8	28.1	5.6	11.4
1962	2154	4230	13.6	26.8	5.4	10.6
1963	2176	4223	13.4	26.1	5.5	10.7
1964	2433	4302	14.3	25.2	5.9	10.4
1965	2574	4356	14.2	24.0	5.8	9.8
1966	2600	4107	14.2	22.4	5.8	9.1
1967	2997	4461	14.4	21.4	5.6	8.4
1968	2913	4225	14.0	20.4	5.3	7.7
1969	3043	4312	13.8	19.6	5.2	7.4
1970	3087	4021	13.8	18.0	4.9	6.4
1971	3055	3546	14.1	16.4	5.0	5.8
1972	3045	3510	14.0	16.2	5.1	5.8
1973	3266	3410	14.4	15.0	5.2	5.5
1974	3253	3467	15.3	16.3	4.8	5.1
1975	3361	3401	15.6	15.8	4.8	4.9
1976	3642	3430	17.0	16.0	5.2	4.8
1977	3390	3633	15.6	16.6	4.8	5.1
1978	3487	3462	15.4	15.2	4.9	4.8
1979	3676	3422	14.6	13.5	4.9	4.5
1980	3691	3363	14.1	12.7	4.7	4.2
1981	3865	3557	14.0	12.6	4.7	4.3
1982	3971	3539	13.5	12.3	4.7	4.2
1983	4077	3586	14.1	12.3	4.7	4.1
1984	4153	3689	14.0	12.4	4.7	4.1
1985	4281	3786	13.9	12.2	4.6	4.0
1986	4237	3877	13.0	11.9	4.5	4.1
1987	4149	3900	14.4	13.5	4.3	4.0

a.   Tax Yields include excise and VAT receipts.

Source: National Income and Expenditure Accounts.

government receipts. By 1987 the yield was only 13 per cent of total tax on expenditure and only 4 per cent of total central government receipts. Whilst the relative importance of alcohol and tobacco taxation as a source of government revenue has declined over the period since 1960, these products remain important sources of tax revenue. Increased tax rates for some categories of these commodities may raise more revenue (such outcomes depend on the value of tax-price elasticities discussed in Chapter 2) but international obligations may inhibit the vigorous use of tax policies which generate both more revenue and less consumption.

CONCLUSION

During the period since 1960 expenditure (deflated to take account of inflation) and volume measures of alcohol consumption both show substantial increases. In terms of litres of pure alcohol per capita of population aged 15 years and over, the consumption of alcohol has increased by 60 per cent.

The market shares of the alcohol products have changed significantly. The levels of expenditure on beer, spirits and wine/perry/cider all show large increases. This development has been accompanied by a reduction in market shares of beer (especially) and spirits (less so) as wine consumption has increased rapidly.

The altered form of alcohol consumption is related closely to relative prices and tax policy. Beer prices have been increased more rapidly than those of spirits and wine and this will have affected its market share. Indeed EC regulations have led to reductions in wine taxation. Another important influence on the consumption of alcohol has been increased purchasing power. The combined effects of tax-price and income (purchasing power) on total alcohol consumption and the relative market shares of alternative products appear to be very significant. The tobacco market has declined significantly in the period since 1960 both in terms of expenditure and volume. This reduced use of tobacco is correlated with declining real prices which might have been expected to have increased consumption. Increased purchasing power might have also been expected to increase the consumption of tobacco. The fact that, despite strong countervailing economic influences, tobacco consumption has fallen is a testimony to the effectiveness of public education campaigns which have demonstrated the health risks associated with the use of this product.

There have been marked changes in the markets for alcohol and consumption since 1960 with alcohol use and apparent associated harm rising significantly and tobacco use and apparent harm declining but remaining the largest avoidable cause of mortality and morbidity (Maynard, Hardman and Whelan, 1987). The factors affecting consumption of these products and the effects changing market sizes have on the industries will be investigated further in the chapters which follow.

SOURCES OF INFORMATION

Central Statistical Office, Annual Abstract of Statistics, HMSO.

- contains annual data on population, volume consumption and consumers' expenditure, imports and exports, personal disposable income.

- annual, the 1988 edition, published in January/February, contains data up to 1986.

Central Statistical Office, Monthly Digest of Statistics, HMSO.

- contains annual and monthly data on volume consumption, imports and exports, personal disposable income, consumers' expenditure.

- monthly publication containing data to 3 months before publication.

Central Statistical Office, United Kingdom National Accounts, HMSO.

- contains data on consumers' expenditure and tax revenues.

- annual, the 1987 edition, published November, contains data up to 1986.

Department of Employment, Employment Gazette, HMSO.

- contains data on retail prices and average earnings.

- monthly publication containing data to 3 months before publication.

The Brewers Society, Statistical Handbook, Brewing Publications Limited, London

- contains comprehensive data on alcoholic drink including volume consumption, consumers' expenditure, prices, imports and exports, taxation revenue, tax rates, population, drinking and driving offences, licenced premises.

- annual, the 1988 edition, published mid-year, contains data up to 1987.

OPCS, Cigarette smoking 1972 to 1986, OPCS Monitor SS 88/1, Government Statistical Service, London.

- contains biannual data in the prevalence of smoking and on cigarette consumption patterns.

- published February 1988—will be updated in two years.

Lee, P.N. (ed.), (1976). Statistics of smoking in the United Kingdom, 7th Edition, Tobacco Research Council, London.

- contains data on tobacco consumption up to 1975. For data since 1976 the Tobacco Advisory Council has published annual facts sheets containing basic data on consumption by weight and volume – available February/March for previous year's figures.

Report of the Commissioners of HM Customs and Excise, HMSO.

- contains data on excise rates for all alcohol and tobacco products.

- financial year data published in December, i.e. 1986–87 duty rates published in December 1987.

References

McDonnell, R. & Maynard, A., (1985), 'Counting the cost of alcohol: gaps in epidemiological knowledge', *Community Medicine*, 7, 4–17.
Maynard, A., Hardman, G., Whelan, A., (1987), 'Data Note 9, Measuring the social costs of addictive substances', *British Journal of Addiction*, 82, 701–706.

2 Modelling demand

CHRISTINE GODFREY

Policies to reduce the consumption of alcohol and tobacco must be based upon an accurate understanding of the factors that affect the demand for these commodities. For example, if the importance of price increases is over-estimated, tax changes will not produce the intended reductions in consumption. Understanding the determination of demand involves identifying the factors that influence consumption and obtaining accurate estimates of their effects. It is not sufficient to rely upon simple correlations or upon untested models that might contain unsuspected defects. Chapter 1 contains an examination of the movement over time of a number of different variables that may influence the level of consumption. The purpose of this chapter is to provide a discussion of the various approaches that have been used to model the relationship between these variables and the level of demand.

The literature on empirical demand models contains many conflicting results and these conflicts have been cited by governments as a reason for inaction; see, for example, a review of the debate of evidence on the effects of advertising on tobacco consumption (Godfrey, 1986a). Health and trade lobbies have both been active in promoting preferred sets of results to support their own viewpoint. Thus there is a clear need to provide a discussion of the differences between alternative approaches and also a framework for evaluating empirical models. Without such a framework, the conflicts between the results for the competing models cannot be resolved and the

35

consequent absence of reliable information is an impediment to the implementation of prevention policies.

The issues involved in describing the current state of the art in modelling demand and in devising statistical methods for detecting inadequate models are of necessity somewhat technical. No attempt will be made to provide full details, but instead emphasis will be placed on communicating the essential features of the problem.

The contents of this chapter are as follows. Individual factors that have been thought to influence the demand for alcohol and tobacco are discussed in the first section, as is their policy relevance. In the second section, the theoretical basis of demand models is examined along with the criteria available to evaluate the different models. In the third section, some results from recent UK studies are reviewed and new empirical estimates are presented. These results are used in Chapter 3 in a discussion of the effects of tax policies. Other prevention policies such as advertising, regulation and health information programmes are considered in the second volume of this series of books.

INDIVIDUAL VARIABLES: DATA CONSTRUCTION AND POLICY RELEVANCE

Previously estimated models vary not only in the variables they have included but also in the way the variables have been measured. The measurement of the most widely used variables is now considered and comments are made upon their relevance for prevention policies.

Consumption

As discussed in Chapter 1, there are a number of different ways of measuring consumption: by expenditure or by volume. Different measures of consumption of alcohol and tobacco have not been perfectly correlated and so results will vary with the choice of consumption measure (see for example Atkinson and Skegg, 1973 for a comparison of alternative measures of tobacco consumption).

The choice of consumption measure depends in part upon the focus of the study. Expenditure series may be appropriate when demand is being estimated for business purposes. In contrast, if the harmful aspects of consumption are of primary interest, then quantity measures such as units of pure alcohol, number of cigarettes, or weight of tobacco may be selected. Any measure may be affected by quality changes, e.g. a switch from high to low tar cigarettes. In order to remove the influence of population size, aggregate consumption measures are usually divided by the number of people over 15 years of age to obtain per capita figures.

No single measure of consumption is accepted as being generally superior to the others and some studies have presented results based upon two or more measures.

Price and income

Specifications of price terms have differed between studies. Some models have used relative or real own price, i.e. own price divided by some index of other prices, but others (e.g. Duffy, 1983) have own price and other prices entered separately. In constructing relative prices, either the Retail Price Index (RPI) or the implicit price deflators described in Chapter 1 have been adopted and generally these series move in line with one another. Some researchers (e.g. Walsh, 1982) have included prices of closely related goods to measure cross price effects, such as the effects of variations in beer price on the consumption of spirits. There has been less variation in the choice of income terms. Most studies have used figures for personal disposable income for the income measure.

An important determinant of own price is tax and tax rates are a policy instrument for influencing consumption and the level of revenue. Income, unlike own price, is not a specific policy variable that can be directly controlled to adjust the levels of alcohol and tobacco consumption. Movements of income may, however, limit the effectiveness of tax changes. The effects of rising incomes on consumption of alcohol and tobacco may offset those of price increases resulting from tax changes.

Advertising

The effect of advertising on consumption has been widely disputed (Godfrey, 1986a). An individual firm will undertake advertising to increase demand for their products and the controversy has surrounded the question as to whether advertising only alters brand shares of the good in question or is capable of increasing the total demand for the good. This is essentially an empirical question and many studies have included an advertising term. The specification and measurement of advertising used has varied between studies.

One measure of advertising is current advertising expenditure (e.g. Witt and Pass, 1981). Others have specified a volume measure of advertising (e.g. McGuinness and Cowling, 1975). Empirical work is limited, however, by the lack of advertising data. In the UK some data are available on press and TV advertising expenditure but, although these constitute the bulk of firms' advertising, the size of the remainder (including posters and cinemas) is not available. It is less clear whether other activities such as sports sponsorship or other marketing expenditure should be included in demand models and, therefore, the lack of data on these activities is probably less important.

Another type of advertising effect was used by Duffy (1983). He included in his study of the demand for alcohol not only a variable measuring advertising on the product in question, but also a variable measuring advertising on all other commodities. The latter variable is predicted to have a negative effect on demand. Thus, for example, the model suggests that if advertising on goods other than beer increases and all other relevant variables are held constant, then the demand for beer will fall.

Health education

Although health education effects have not been included in models of alcohol demand, most empirical work of tobacco demand has included a measure of health education. In general, these studies have specified some shock effect occurring with major events such as the publication of the first and subsequent reports by the Royal College of Physicians (RCP). There have, however, been considerable variations in details of the specification of health education effects. Atkinson and Skegg (1973) and Witt and Pass (1981) specified models in which, after initial shocks, consumption would return to previous levels, other things being equal. In the former study, this return was assumed to be gradual whereas in the latter it occurred instantly after a prespecified period, e.g. two years. McGuinness and Cowling (1975) did not allow for a return to previous levels of consumption, but instead regarded health publicity as having a specific anti-advertising effect.

Although more complex specifications of health effects may be of interest, estimating the health education impact will still involve considerable measurement problems and such models are unlikely to be capable of providing a complete evaluation of the impact of any one education campaign.

Licensing and other regulations

The retailing of alcohol has historically been subject to considerable regulation. Liberalisation of the licensing laws has been criticised by many of those worried about increasing alcohol abuse. It is therefore perhaps surprising that demand models for alcohol have not always considered a variable measuring the influence of alcohol availability. The link between the number of licenses and overall consumption is, however, not straightforward.

If licensing laws restrict the number of available outlets, then this obviously affects suppliers, but may not necessarily affect demand directly.

Indirect effects may occur if the licensing laws restrict competition: prices may be higher or public houses may offer fewer services. Two arguments have been proposed for a direct effect on demand. A restricted number of outlets may increase transaction costs, e.g. travel to outlets etc, and thereby reduce demand. Also the outlets (and posters or logos near them) may act as advertising stimulating demand. In three major UK studies, McGuinness (1980) and Duffy (1980, 1983) have taken different views on the direction of the causality between the number of licensed outlets and the consumption of alcohol. McGuinness considered that the length of time preceding the opening of new licensed premises ruled out the possibility of current demand influencing the number of licensed premises. He included licensing variables in his study and hypothesised that there were no feedback effects between licensing and demand. In contrast, Duffy (1983) argued that the growth in sales determined licences, but the number of licences had no effect on demand. In the third section results are reported from an investigation of the possibility of feedback effects (see Godfrey, 1988). Such investigation is important because the statistical methods usually employed are invalid when feedback effects exist and will produce biased estimates.

Tobacco retailing is not subject to the same degree of regulation as alcohol, retailing licensing law being abolished in 1962. As with alcohol, retailing of tobacco has undergone considerable changes. The promotion of loss leaders, including the discounting of large quantities of cigarettes, is likely to directly affect demand through changes in price and the number of outlets is probably not needed as a separate variable in the demand equation. Although no UK study has attempted to measure the effect of the number of outlets on cigarette demand, Yucelt and Kaynak (1984) did include such a variable in their analysis of US data. Their results indicated that this variable was not significant in any of their model specifications.

Licensing of outlets is only one regulatory control. US studies have considered a number of other measures such as the impact of minimum drinking ages (see for example Saffer and Grossman, 1987). Special data are needed for such studies and have usually been unavailable to fully evaluate changes in policy that have been enacted in the UK such as the Scottish licensing law changes.

DEMAND MODELS AND THEIR EVALUATION

Different models of demand

The empirical demand models that have featured in the literature and policy debates have differed in a number of ways. These differences are reflected in variations in results that make it difficult to form a clear assessment of the impact of prevention policies. It is useful to divide the discussion of the differences into four parts: the choice of functional form to approximate the actual demand relationship; the type of data used in the estimation of the statistical model; the theoretical underpinning of the statistical model; and the treatment of habit formation. This discussion covers some relatively technical issues, but they cannot be ignored. Many models may be fitted to various sets of data. However, without an understanding of their limitations and the criteria by which they should be judged, it is all too easy to obtain a wide range of conflicting results that are of little real value in the investigation of the likely effects of prevention policies.

Functional form Economic theory suggests variables that may be expected to influence the demand for a commodity, but usually offers little guidance about the precise mathematical form of the relationship. This mathematical form is needed for statistical analysis. Functional forms are often selected after consideration of ease of estimation and interpretation. The most widely used form are the linear and doubly logarithmic specification. A linear relationship between two variables x and y, can be written as

$$y = a + b\,x,$$

where a and b are coefficients, with the doubly logarithmic version being

$$\log(y) = a' + b'\log(x).$$

where a' and b' are coefficients.

In order to compare results derived using different specifications, economists have adopted a unit free index known as the elasticity. A price elasticity can be defined as follows. If price changes by a small amount, with all other variables that influence demand being held constant, then demand will also change: the price elasticity is defined as the ratio of the proportionate change in demand to the proportionate change in price. Roughly speaking, an own price elasticity for tobacco of –0.5, would imply that a 1 per cent increase in the price of cigarettes, with all other factors being fixed, would lead to a 0.5 per cent drop in the demand for cigarettes. Income and other elasticities (e.g. advertising) can be defined in a similar way and an income elasticity for cigarettes of 0.7 would suggest that a 1 per cent increase in income would be accompanied by a 0.7 per cent increase in the demand for cigarettes.

In the doubly logarithmic functional form, elasticities are constant over the whole range of observations but this is not always a plausible assumption. So, for example, as incomes rise the demand for relatively expensive goods such as spirits might be expected to become less responsive to price. Other functional forms do not have constant elasticities. The price elasticities, for example in a linear model, depend upon the price level. In the absence of other information, functional form must be selected using statistical criteria as part of the testing procedure to establish that a model is consistent with the data.

Types of data   Data availability is an important constraint on the type of models that can be estimated. In recent years the increasing availability of individual or household surveys such as the Family Expenditure Survey (FES) or General Household Survey (GHS) has widened the type of analyses that can be undertaken (see Atkinson, Gomulka and Stern, 1986a, 1986b; Jones, 1987). With data on individuals, sociological and other variables thought to influence consumption habits can be introduced. Also by considering different price and income responses over different groups of individuals, such as rich and poor, male and female, heavy or light consumers, the differential effects of policy and the consequences of policy can be investigated. Measures of alcohol and tobacco consumption obtained from budget and other surveys have, however, been criticised on the grounds of reliability. When compared to the national account estimates, the extent of under-reporting in the FES has been calculated at 22 to 26 per cent for tobacco and 40 to 45 per cent for alcohol (see Atkinson, Gomulka and Stern, 1984a, 1984b; Kemsley, Redpath and Holmes, 1980). Any projections from such sample survey to the whole population, have, therefore, to be considered with care.

The availability and accuracy of time series data are in part responsible for the large number of studies that attempt to describe the changing consumption of alcohol or tobacco products over a number of years. Models using these data, therefore, assume that the demand relationships are aggregated over individuals, or can be regarded as representative of an individual.

In this series of books, we are concentrating on national prevention policies and their effects on the overall level of consumption. Provided they are adequate approximations, time series models are particularly useful for policy simulations concerning aggregate consumption, and such models have formed the majority of the existing studies. The following analyses, therefore, concentrate on models using time series data.

Different types of theoretical model   Two distinct approaches have emerged in estimating demand for different goods. The most common assumption is to consider the demand for any one good in isolation, i.e. the single equation approach. Such equations only include price terms of a few close substitutes (or complements) and/or represent the effect of all other prices by some composite index. The approach has little theoretical foundation and therefore careful testing of empirical results is important.

Single equation studies have varied in the assumptions made about the appropriate level of product aggregation. Both alcohol and tobacco contain a number of different constituent parts. Cigarettes, cigars and pipe tobacco are all tobacco products. The variety of alcohol products is wide and even within the main groups (beer, spirits and wine) there are many different products. Some studies have used a very broad definition of all alcohol. Estimating similar models using different levels of aggregation in construction of variables can produce different results. For example, after McGuinness (1980) estimated a demand model for all alcohol, Walsh (1982) re-estimated the model using separate equations for beer, spirits and wine and obtained results which were quite unlike those reported by McGuinness.

The second approach involves estimating complete systems of demand equations. The demand system approach is designed to consider the interrelationships between goods and could be valuable in considering a number of policy changes. It would be useful, for example, to estimate what would be substituted in consumers' budgets if policies were successful in reducing the demand for cigarettes.

There are, however, problems with this second approach. Its assumptions are often found to be inconsistent with the sample evidence and no specification of the various demand systems that have been proposed has emerged as the 'best' model. It is, however, interesting to note that cross-price effects, e.g. the impact on wine consumption of an increase in the price of beer, have usually been found to be small (see Duffy, 1987; Salvananthan, 1985). Barten (1975) and Deaton and Meullbauer (1980) provide an assessment of previous empirical estimates.

Dynamic and habit forming specifications   It is often argued that the consumption of tobacco and alcohol is habit forming. Consequently some empirical work has addressed the problem of taking account of dynamics and habit effects. Much of this work stems from the pioneering analysis of Houthakker and Taylor (1970) and variants of their model have been used for demand studies of types of alcohol and tobacco consumption.

Houthakker and Taylor related demand not only to price and income, but also to a variable measuring the existing stocks of the commodity. For goods such as alcohol and tobacco, Houthakker and Taylor considered that the stock measure could be viewed as a psychological stock variable, measuring habit formation and inertia. In this case, the coefficient of the stock variable should be positive, i.e. the more the consumer drank/smoked in the past, the more he will want to drink/smoke now.

Empirical results for this model have been mixed. Duffy (1980) found that the estimated parameters were outside the acceptable range when he estimated the model for beer, wines and spirits. For example, his estimates suggested that past drinking depressed current consumption. Kennedy et al. (1973) using Irish data came to a more positive conclusion on the usefulness of the dynamic specification. Tsolakis, Reithmuller and Watts (1983) also found this model compatible with Australian wine consumption, but its application to beer consumption was less successful.

Another model that has been used, particularly for cigarette consumption, is the partial adjustment model. The desired level of consumption is a function of prices, income and other factors, but a variety of circumstances prevent consumers fully adjusting to this desired level in the period. Actual consumption is then assumed to be a weighted average of desired and past consumption. This form has been the basis of many of the demand studies (e.g. McGuinness and Cowling, 1975; Metra, 1979).

The use of this model for modelling cigarette or tobacco consumption has, however, been criticised by Johnston (1980) who suggested that the partial adjustment model is appropriate for situations where the cost of adjustment (e.g. financial, legal or institutional) is high, but that there is no reason for this to be the case for cigarettes or tobacco consumption. Duffy (1980) suggested that this argument also holds for alcohol consumption. Another interpretation of the importance of lagged consumption is that it is indirectly measuring the effect of past consumption levels influencing present levels (Brown, 1952).

A third group of models involving habit effects takes as its basis the hypothesis that consumers may respond asymmetrically to changes in market forces. In particular, for substances like tobacco and alcohol, consumers may have a tendency to acquire a habit more easily at times of low prices or high income, and be reluctant to abandon them when prices rise and income falls. So, for example, considering price changes only, the response to a price rise would be smaller than to a price fall of the same amount.

Young's (1983) analysis of such a model using US data indicated that this phenomenon has important policy implications. Whereas an analysis assuming symmetric responses to prices had yielded the result that tax changes leading to a price rise of 10 per cent would lower consumption by 4.5 per cent, Young's estimates indicate that a price rise of 14 per cent would be required to obtain the same reduction in consumption. A fuller analysis and review of these models and other issues discussed in this chapter is given in Godfrey (1986b).

Evaluating competing models

The brief survey above suggests that there are a number of competing models that can be used to estimate the demand for alcohol and tobacco. With little theoretical guidance as to the correct specification, it is especially important to evaluate the adequacy of empirical studies in order to separate the wheat from the chaff. Recent work in the field of the statistical testing of economic models has suggested the development of some minimal statistical criteria by which to judge the adequacy of models (see Hendry, 1983).

The process of assessing the adequacy of empirical models can be thought of as having two parts: first, to check whether or not the assumptions of that model are consistent with the observed data; and second, to investigate whether or not the model can account for the results obtained using competing specifications.

Investigation of a model's ability to encompass the results of competing relationships can be conducted by forming a comprehensive model against which the model of interest is tested. (A comprehensive model is one that includes all competing specifications as special cases.) The idea of nesting a model in a more general comprehensive specification is perhaps more familiar to applied workers, and fortunately many of the specifications used to estimate tobacco demand can be regarded as special cases of Young's (1983) model. The general Young model of tobacco demand has been subjected to a number of tests to determine whether simplifications are acceptable (see Godfrey, 1986c). The models of Duffy (1983) and McGuinness (1983) have also been evaluated using statistical tests (see Godfrey, 1988).

The use of statistical tests provides a systematic way of assessing the performance of different models. Some caution must be adopted in considering the results of studies which have not used such techniques as they may suffer from misspecifications that invalidate the estimates and may lead to misleading results.

COMPARISON OF EMPIRICAL RESULTS

In this section we discuss some of the findings from previous work and then present results from two studies (Godfrey, 1986c and 1988) which have attempted to evaluate the models using statistical techniques. Alcohol and tobacco studies are considered separately, and the implications of the results for prevention policy examined.

Tobacco

Investigations of the factors that influence cigarette and tobacco consumption have prompted a number of debates about the effects of alternative government prevention policies. Many of the earlier studies (e.g. Sumner, 1971; Atkinson and Skegg, 1973; Russell, 1973; Peto, 1974) were concerned with comparing the merits of tax increases and health education policies as instruments for reducing the level of tobacco consumption. Later work (e.g. McGuinness and Cowling, 1975; the Metra Report, 1979) concentrated on the effects of advertising on consumption.

Table 2.1
Price elasticity estimates

Study	Data	Elasticities
RUSSELL (1973)	1946–1971 (annual)	−0.5 to −0.66
ATKINSON AND SKEGG (1973)	1951–1970 (annual)	0.0 (men) −0.35 (women)
SUMNER (1972)	1955–1968	−0.8
PETO (1974)	1951–1970 (annual)	−0.37 to −0.64 (men)
McGUINESS AND COWLING (1975)	1957–1968 (annual)	SR −0.99 LR −1.05
WITT AND PASS (1981)	1955–1975 (annual)	−0.32
METRA (1979)	1958–1978 (quarterly)	SR −0.32 to −0.54 LR −0.42 to −0.54
RADFAR (1985)	1965–1980 (quarterly)	SR −0.23 LR −0.39

SR = short run, LR = long run

Source: Godfrey and Maynard (1988)

Price and income elasticities calculated from these early studies are presented in Tables 2.1 and 2.2. Estimates of price elasticity vary considerably with very low estimates of price elasticity reported by Atkinson and Skegg (1973), and much higher estimates obtained by McGuinness and Cowling (1975). Such differences in estimates would imply quite different changes in price to achieve, for example, a 10 per cent change in consumption. Income elasticities shown in Table 2.2 have, in general, shown less variation.

Table 2.2

Income elasticity estimates

Study	Elasticities
ATKINSON AND SKEGG	0.36
PETO (1974)	−0.14 to −0.49
McGUINESS AND COWLING (1975)	SR −0.31 LR 0.12
WITT AND PASS (1981)	−0.13
RADFAR (1985)	SR −0.12 LR −0.19

SR = short run, LR = long run
Source: Godfrey and Maynard (1988)

Not all the studies included an advertising term and the few studies that did, McGuinness and Cowling (1975), Metra (1979), Radfar (1985) and Witt and Pass (1981), had conflicting findings. From McGuinness and Cowling's study, a long run advertising elasticity was calculated at 0.09. A short run elasticity of 0.09 and a long run elasticity of 0.15 were found when Radfar re-estimated the McGuinness and Cowling model. Witt and Pass (1981), using different models and data, also found statistically significant advertising effects and calculated an advertising elasticity of 0.07. On the other hand Metra, in a study commissioned by two tobacco companies, found no significant advertising effects.

One factor of special interest in examining the determinants of tobacco consumption is the effect of health education. The specification of health education effects has varied as described in the previous sections. In some models health education shocks have been specified as having a permanent effect in reducing consumption, others have assumed that such effects are of a limited duration. Earlier studies had indicated sizeable effects. Sumner (1971) estimated that the 1962 Report of the Royal College of Physicians decreased consumption by 2 per cent for each year up to the end of his data period 1967. Atkinson and Skegg (1973) estimated that the 1962 RCP report, the 1965 television advertising ban on cigarettes and the 1971 RCP report each reduced consumption by 5 per cent, but this effect died away at 1 per cent per annum. Witt and Pass (1981) also specified models incorporating a limited duration of health effects. McGuinness and Cowling (1975) and Radfar (1985) found health education shocks reduced advertising elasticities.

In summary, therefore, this brief review of empirical work indicates a number of differences in reported results. Moreover, the current relevance of these results is open to question because there has been a large decrease in consumption, and large variations in tobacco prices and disposable income since 1975. In order to obtain results using post 1975 data, a number of models employing annual observations for the period 1956–84 have been estimated and evaluated (Godfrey, 1986c). It was found that, in general, the Young (1983) model described above passed tests for misspecification. As expected, estimates of individual coefficients varied with the choice of consumption measure and the specification of health education effects.

The price elasticity of –0.56 implied by one of the models is larger than some previous estimates given in Table 2.1, but is close to the Treasury estimate of –0.5 (as is the income elasticity). Another interesting feature of this model is that it implies a continual 3 per cent fall in demand per annum after the effect of the first health shock of 1962, rather than a return to previous levels of consumption.

Significant advertising coefficients were found in some specifications, with short run elasticities being of a similar magnitude (0.11 to 0.07) to those of earlier studies. The specification of the health effects had a considerable effect on the results of the model and new specifications may be worth exploring.

In addition to health education effects, there are several other areas that require further research if reliable models are to be obtained to examine policy measures. One suggestion is that participation and consumption decisions should be considered separately (Jones, 1986). Unfortunately there are no consistent annual series of the participation rates, so that there are considerable data problems.

Also it may be useful to consider difficult groups separately. The disaggregated studies that have been undertaken, such as Atkinson and Skegg (1973) and Townsend (1987), suggest that effects of price and other variables may vary between different groups. Such disaggregated studies, however, need a rich data set which is sometimes difficult to acquire. Atkinson and Skegg, for example, used data published by the Tobacco Advisory Council (TAC). Although the TAC supplied data on the different rates of male and female smoking to the last RCP report, the data are no longer published. General Household Survey data are only collected biannually and therefore smoking data are only available for a limited number of data points.

Alcohol

Three recent studies are to be considered, namely those of McGuinness (1983), Walsh (1982) and Duffy (1983). There were some similarities between these studies, e.g. all three presented separate equations for beer, spirits and wine, but there are important differences in many aspects of the empirical analyses.

Duffy argued that not only did licensing effects play no role in determining consumption, but that in fact consumption levels influenced the number of licensed premises. Duffy's argument implies that the other two studies include an irrelevant variable and, perhaps more importantly, that their estimates may be affected by feedback bias.

Given the various differences between the data and model specifications of the three different studies under consideration, it is not surprising that there is some variation in their results. These results can be compared using the estimates given in Table 2.3. This table reports the estimates of own price and income elasticities reported in the studies. The table also contains the estimated elasticities used by the Treasury in revenue calculations (HM Treasury, 1982).

Table 2.3

Own price and income elasticities of earlier studies

	Beer		Spirits		Wine		Time period
	Own price	Income	Own price	Income	Own price	Income	of study
Walsh	Vol −0.13	0.13	−0.47	1.20	−0.28	0.51	1955–1975
	Exp −0.26	0.12	−0.45	0.99	−0.38	0.49	(annual)
McGuinness	−0.30	0.13	−0.38	1.54	−0.17	1.11	1956–1979
							(annual)
Duffy	Not available	0.8 to 1.1	−0.8 to −1.0	1.6	−0.7 to −1.0	2.2 to 2.5	1963–1978 (quarterly)
Treasury	−0.5	−0.55	−1.3	1.75	−1.3	2.6 (Light wine)	
					−1.6	2.0 (Other wine)	
					−0.5	0.5 (Cider)	

Source: Godfrey 1986b and Treasury estimates from personal communication.

Given the recent debates on the role of advertising, it is interesting to note that all three studies found little evidence of large advertising effects. McGuinness' results are a mixture of significant and insignificant coefficients and, in his own words '... do not suggest that small changes in the levels of real advertising of alcohol will have much of an effect on consumption levels'.

A licensing variable was used in only two of the alcohol studies, namely those of McGuinness and Walsh. Both researchers found that the number of licences had significant coefficients in the beer equation and the estimated coefficient was also large in McGuinness' results. Moreover, in Walsh's estimates, the licences variable was also significant in the spirits and wine equations. Such results may be felt to give some support to those who have been concerned about the effect of growth in the number of licensed premises.

It was the role of the licensing variable which was the focus of an econometric analysis (Godfrey, 1988). A set of statistical tests as used in an attempt to detect unsound models that might lead to misleading conclusions. Test procedures were applied to models for each type of alcoholic drink in turn. For beer expenditure and volume, feedback effects between licensing and consumption were found for all the specifications, thus providing some support for at least part of Duffy's argument and casting doubt upon the results reported in previous research. For spirits and wine, whether measured in expenditure or volume terms, there was no evidence of a feedback effect between licensing and demand. The omission of licensing effects was consistent with the data for most of the specifications of spirits consumption models. For wine consumption, the results for the volume measure suggested that there was a significant licensing effect with estimated elasticities ranging from 1.39 to 4.94. An elasticity value of 1.39 would suggest that a 10 per cent fall in the number of licensed outlets per adult would be accompanied by a 13.9 per cent fall in wine consumption.

Table 2.4

Price and income elasticities for wines and spirits (evaluated for 1980)

	Nominal Own price (Duffy model)	Relative own price (McGuiness model)	Income
Spirits expenditure	−1.07, −3.03	−0.61 to −0.82	1.39 to 2.09
Spirits volume	−0.88, −0.98	−0.56 to −0.99	0.6 to 2.76
Wine expenditure	−2.67	−0.26 to −0.63	1.25 to 1.70
Wine volume	−0.76[a], −1.14[a]	−0.91[a]	1.10 to 1.70

a. Based on statistically insignificant coefficients.

Source: Godfrey (1988).

Income and own price elasticities for spirits and wine calculated 1980 data are given in Table 2.4. Although price and income were generally found to be important determinants of wine and spirits consumption, the sample data were consistent with a wide range of estimates. It is difficult to choose a particular set of values for policy simulations of, for example, a tax change.

Overall, a general point that emerged was that with the limited data available it is not always possible to detect inadequate models by means of standard statistical tests. Consequently, care should be exercised when interpreting the results of an empirical study. The fact that tests may lack power in detecting misspecification does not, of course, imply that they should be ignored. Without such checks, situations may arise in which policy recommendations are based upon grossly misspecified models and misleading results.

CONCLUSION

The empirical analysis of demand models has indicated that economic variables do affect the consumption of alcohol and tobacco, although the estimates of the exact magnitudes of their effects have varied from one study to another. As far as prevention policy is concerned, one of the key variables influencing demand is price because it can be manipulated using tax changes. For tobacco, a price elasticity of about –0.5 to –0.6 is suggested by empirical work. An elasticity of –0.5 would imply that price would have to be increased by 20 per cent to achieve a 10 per cent reduction in consumption. Smaller price increases would be required if tax changes were supported by a continuing health education effort. Controlling alcohol consumption by means of tax changes is a complex problem because the price elasticities for different types of alcoholic beverages vary substantially. There is general agreement that the consumption of beer is not very responsive to changes in its price although the Treasury has recently revised its elasticity estimate from –0.2 to –0.5. For spirits and wine, estimates are more varied but indicate a greater degree of price sensitivity. Controls on the number of licensed outlets may be useful to restrict consumption of wine, with estimates suggesting that a 15 per cent reduction in the number of licensed outlets per adult might provide a 20 per cent fall in wine consumption.

It is, however, hazardous to predict mechanically responses to substantial policy changes using past empirical work. For both alcohol and tobacco, the limitations of empirical study may be considerable and are not always obvious. There are dangers in using untested models based upon out-of-date data for predicting the effects of alternative policies. Even if new models with improved and extended data sets are judged to be adequate and provide plausible results, not all effects may be precisely estimated. Moreover, statistical significance should not be confused with some idea of major quantitative importance of a variable. Nor is it necessarily possible to forecast the effect of new policies from models estimated with past data. Such models should only be expected to forecast small changes in variables with accuracy. Clearly a policy event, such as an advertising ban, is outside the range of currently observed data and may have effects above those predicted for zero expenditure using estimates calculated from that data. Similarly the effects of a major health advertising campaign could not be evaluated accurately from existing models of the health education effects.

Notwithstanding these cautious comments, well-constructed and tested demand models represent a method of increasing knowledge about smoking and drinking behaviour. Although conclusions from these models are limited by the problems of interpretation and model comparison discussed in this chapter, they can provide valuable information to assist the process of policy formation.

References

Atkinson, A.B., Gomulka, J. and Stern, N.M., (1984a), Household Expenditure on Tobacco 1970–1980: Evidence from the Family Expenditure Surveys, ESRC Programme on Taxation, Incentives and the Distribution of Income, Working Paper No. 57.

Atkinson, A.B., Gomulka, J. and Stern, M., (1984b), Expenditure on Alcohol Drink by Households: Evidence from the Family Expenditure Survey, 1970–1980, ESRC Programme on Taxation, Incentives and the Distribution of Income, Discussion Paper 60.

Atkinson, A.B. and Skegg, J.L., (1973), 'Anti-smoking publicity and the demand for tobacco in the UK', *The Manchester School*, 41, 265–282.

Barten, A.P., (1975), The systems of consumer demand functions approach: a review, in Intriligator, M.D. (ed.) *Frontiers of Quantitative Economics*, Vol. 2, 355–71.

Deaton and Meullbauer, (1980), *Economics and Consumer Behaviour*, Cambridge University Press, Cambridge.

Duffy, M., (1980), Advertising, Taxation and the Demand for Beer, Spirits and Wine in the United Kingdom 1963–78, Occasional Paper No. 8009, Department of Management Sciences, UMIST.

Duffy, M., (1983), 'The demand for alcoholic drink in the United Kingdom', 1963–78, *Applied Economics*, 15, 125–140.

Duffy, M., (1987), 'Advertising and the inter-product distribution of demand: a Rotterdam model approach', *European Economic Review*, 31 (5), 1051–1070.

Godfrey, C., (1986a), 'Government policy, advertising and tobacco consumption in the UK: a critical review of the literature', *British Journal of Addiction*, 81, 339–346.

Godfrey, C., (1986b), Factors Influencing the Consumption of Alcohol and Tobacco - a review of demand models, *Centre for Health Economics, Discussion Paper 17*, University of York.

Godfrey, C., (1986c), Price and advertising elasticities of the demand for tobacco, Working Paper, ESRC Addiction Research Centre, University of York.

Godfrey, C., (1988), 'Licensing and the demand for alcohol', *Applied Economics*, 20, 1541–1558.

Godfrey, C. and Maynard, A., (1988), 'Economic aspects of tobacco use and taxation policy', *British Medical Journal*, 297, 339–343.

Hendry, D.F., (1983), 'Econometric modelling: the consumption function in retrospect', *Scottish Journal of Political Economy*, 30, 193– 220.

HM Treasury, (1982), Macroeconomic Model of Technical Manual, HM Treasury, London.

Houthakker, H.S. and Taylor, L.D., (1970), *Consumer Demand in the United States*, Harvard University Press, Cambridge, Massachusetts, USA.

Johnston, J., (1980), 'Advertising and the aggregate demand for cigarettes: a comment', *European Economic Review*, 14, 117–125.

Jones, A., (1986), The economics of addiction - a dual approach, Paper presented to the Health Economists Study Group, York, 8–10 January 1986

Jones, A., (1987), A double hurdle model of cigarette consumption. IRISS, Department of Economics Discussion Paper 128, University of York.

Kemsley, W.W.F., Redpath, R.U. and Holmes, M., (1980), *Family Expenditure Survey Handbook*, HMSO, London.

Kennedy, K.A., Ebrill, L. and Walsh, B.M., (1973), The Demand for Beer and Spirits in Ireland, *Proceedings of the Royal Irish Academy*, 73, Section C, No. 13.

McGuinness, T., (1980), 'An econometric analysis of total demand for alcoholic beverages in the UK, 1956–1975', *Journal of Industrial Economics*, September, 85–109.

McGuinness, T., (1983), 'The Demand for Beer, Spirits and Wine in the UK, 1956–1979', in Grant, M., Plant, M. and Williams, A. (eds.), *Economics and Alcohol*, Croom Helm, London.

McGuinness, T. and Cowling, K., (1975), 'Advertising and the aggregate demand for cigarettes', *European Economic Review*, 6, 311–328.

Metra Consulting Group Limited, (1979), *The Relationship between Total Cigarette Advertising and Total Cigarette Consumption in the UK*, Metra, London.

Peto, J., (1974), 'Price and consumption of cigarettes: a case for intervention', *British Journal of Social and Preventive Medicine*, 28, 241–245.

Radfar, M., (1985), 'The effect of advertising on total consumption of cigarettes in the UK', *European Economic Review*, 29, 225–231.

Royal College of Physicians, (1962), *Smoking and Health*, Pitman, London.

Russell, M.A., (1973), 'Changes in cigarette price and consumption by men in Britain 1946–1974', *British Journal of Preventive and Social Medicine*, 27, No.1.

Saffer, H. and Grossman, M., (1987), 'Drinking age laws and highway mortality rates: cause and effect', *Economic Inquiry*, 25, 403– 477.

Selvanathan, E.A., (1985), The Demand for Alcohol in the UK: An Econometric Study. Discussion Paper 85.06, Department of Economics, The University of Western Australia.

Sumner, M.T., (1971), 'Demand for tobacco in the UK', *The Manchester School*, 39, 23–36.

Townsend, J., (1987), 'Cigarette tax, economic welfare and social class patterns of smoking', *Applied Economics*, 19, 355–365.

Tsolakis, D., Reithmuller, P. and Watts, G., (1983), 'The demand for wine and beer', *Review of Marketing and Agricultural Economics*, 51(2), 131–153.

Walsh, B.M., (1982), 'The demand for alcohol in the UK: a comment', *Journal of Industrial Economics*, 30(4), 439–446.

Witt, S.F. and Pass, C.L., (1981), 'The effects of health warnings and advertising on the demand for cigarettes', *Scottish Journal of Political Economy*, 28, 86–91.

Young, T., (1983), 'The demand for cigarettes: alternative specifications of Fujii's model', *Applied Economics*, 15, 203–211.

Yucelt, U. and Kaynak, E., (1984), 'A study of measuring influence of advertising and forecasting cigarette sales', *Managerial and Decision Economics*, 5(4), 213–218.

3 Preventive health objectives and tax policy options

CHRISTINE GODFREY AND LARRY HARRISON

The prices of alcohol and tobacco goods were identified in Chapter 2 as important determinants of their levels of consumption. All alcohol and tobacco goods are subject to high levels of taxation and the level of taxation is a significant influence on the price of these goods. Since increasing the level of taxes may lead to higher prices and lower consumption, tax changes represent a potential preventive health policy available to governments.

Health objectives are, of course, not the only factors that are considered by governments deciding upon tax policy. As indicated by the data presented in Chapter 1, alcohol and tobacco taxes are major sources of revenue and revenue considerations can be expected to play an important role. Also general economic considerations will affect the tax policy decision making process. The purpose of this chapter is to consider what tax options are available to control consumption and whether health and other objectives are incompatible.

Before describing tax policy options, it will be useful to outline the alternative objectives that might underpin them and to examine the potential for conflicts between these objectives. This preliminary discussion provides a framework for the evaluation of policy options and is contained in the first section. It is followed by an examination of policies with health objectives that could be introduced without changes to the present budgetary system. The analysis is then extended by considering a second set of policies that are differentiated by the fact that they would require changes in the budgetary system. Finally, both sets of policies are examined in the light of proposals for EC tax harmonisation.

OBJECTIVES AND PRINCIPLES FOR TAXING ALCOHOL AND TOBACCO

Health campaigners have concentrated on the potential use of tax increases to reduce consumption. An alternative health based policy would be to use tax to reduce the social costs associated with alcohol and tobacco policies. In this section these two health objectives are examined. Considerations relevant to the revenue raising characteristics of alcohol and tobacco are then discussed.

Social cost and prevention objectives

One justification for preventive taxes on alcohol and tobacco is based on the costs associated with the consumption of these products. Policies might be based on so called external costs, i.e. those factors not taken into account by individuals in their consumption decisions and borne unwillingly by others in society. One possible prevention policy is to set a tax on the commodities at a rate at which consumers would choose the same amount as if they had to take all the relevant costs into account. It should be noted that this optimum level of tax need no result in zero levels of harm.

There are problems in implementing an externality type policy. One problem is to identify what constitutes an external cost and how these costs can be measured; see Littlechild and Wiseman (1986) for a discussion of various types of externalities. Most empirical studies have attempted to evaluate total social costs and have not distinguished between those costs borne by the individual smoker or drinker and those borne by the rest of society. Some items of costs, such as loss of life, mental distress or impaired quality of life, are difficult to quantify. Nor do we have sufficient information to estimate the exact relationship between levels of consumption and levels of harm (see Godfrey and Powell, 1987a for a discussion of these issues).

There would be additional problems in introducing such policies. For example, it is possible that these costs increase more than proportionally with consumption. As a result each individual would have to be observed in order to determine the tax rate. Also different groups generate different levels of external costs, e.g. the young compared to the old. It is clearly either impossible or prohibitively costly to conduct monitoring and to have tax rates differentiated by groups and/or past consumption.

Godfrey and Powell (1987b) suggest, however, that despite these problems the theory can be used to provide generalised rules for prevention taxes. Such rules are based on the characteristic of the good that is linked to the external costs. To set taxes it is, however, necessary to identify the connection between consumption and harm. For alcohol this is generally taken to be pure alcohol content. The current system imposes much higher taxes per volume of alcohol on spirits than on other beverages. There is, however, little evidence to suggest that spirits drinkers create greater levels of external costs than other drinkers (Wagenaar, 1984; Perrine, 1975; Berger and Snortum, 1985). One appropriate rule may be, therefore, to equalise tax per unit alcohol both across and within beverage types. The issue of equal tax per unit alcohol is discussed in Chapter 9 in the context of the Scotch whisky industry.

There has been some debate as to the appropriate characteristic for tobacco. Health effects are sometimes linked to the number of cigarettes smoked. The number of cigarettes smoked is, however, likely to be an inadequate indicator because it does not take account of relevant factors; for example, health effects will depend upon whether the cigarette is filter tipped or untipped, is low tar or high tar. Perhaps a better indicator of health effects is the weight of tobacco smoked and Kay and Keen (1982) suggest tobacco weight may be the most relevant characteristic. This measure was the basis of taxation before 1978. Another alternative is to set differential taxes according to tar content. Harris (1980) examined the theory behind the implementation of such a tax and suggested that its validity depended on the relationship of tar content and harm, i.e. does the smoking of a few high tar cigarettes cause the same amount of damage as the equivalent tar level from a larger number of low tar cigarettes. He also suggested that the possible number of different graduations of tax will be determined by administrative costs. It should be noted in this context that such a tax may not be based on pure external costs, for example the effect of passive smoking or fires, but on general health effects. Some economists (Atkinson and Meade, 1974; Leu and Schaub, 1984) have extended the externality model to include private costs (for example costs to the individual of ill health) not valued by consumers because of the lack of information about health risks.

The important conclusion from the consideration of the rules derived from the externality model is that they operate on price rather than consumption. If demand is inelastic, the fall in consumption which results from such a policy may be relatively small (see Chapter 2).

Paternalist or consumption objectives

The externality model is based on the assumption that consumers are able to make rational choices about consuming alcohol and tobacco. Governments may seek to introduce paternalist policies if they believe that some or all consumers are not able to make reasonable decisions (Littlechild and Wiseman, 1986). Many government policies, for example, are framed to protect children. With alcohol and tobacco consumption, additional arguments are raised about dependence or addiction and the inability of consumers to assess risks (see Leu, 1983). It is, however, difficult to assess such arguments within a pure economic efficiency model and to obtain unique targets for policies.

In general, it may be expected that such policies would aim to reduce consumption by some, for example the young, or all consumers by imposing a tax on consumption. In order to control consumption, however, it is necessary to consider the effect of income as well as prices on consumption. This has led to suggestions that tax rates should be indexed to changes in income as well as changes in prices. For smoking, the link between consumption and harm is generally accepted and therefore the aim of such a policy would be to control levels of per capita consumption. For alcohol, a similar policy target of per capita consumption has been based on the association between per capita consumption and indicators of harm (Bruun et al., 1979; Saunders, 1985). Such general relationships do not, however, usually result in agreed safe target levels of per capita consumption and policy recommendations with precise target levels of consumption are rare.

Revenue and other considerations

Governments need revenue for a number of purposes. In raising revenue, however, governments will wish to avoid undesirable economic consequences, and the effects that taxes may have on the welfare of individuals has been the subject of considerable debate. In this section, some of the arguments on the appropriateness of alcohol and tobacco taxes for general revenue raising are considered.

Revenue considerations Revenue and health objectives may conflict if increasing the tax rate on a commodity leads to a decline in revenue. A number of factors determine the relationship between tax changes and revenue yield. First, the manufacturer will decide how much of the tax change to pass on in the form of a price increase. Consumers will then change their consumption in the light of the price increase, and the interaction of all these decisions will lead to a change in tax revenue. Responsiveness of consumption to price and of tax revenue to tax changes are usually discussed

57

in policy studies in terms of elasticities. Elasticities are unit-free measures with, for example, the tax elasticity being (approximately) the percentage change in revenue resulting from a one per cent change in tax rates. The discussion above indicates that this elasticity will depend upon the price elasticity of demand (the consumers' responsiveness to price changes) and, under the assumption that tax changes are passed on in full, the proportion of price represented by tax.

The current Treasury estimates of price elasticities imply that revenue would increase if alcohol and tobacco taxes were increased (see Chapter 2). Consequently the maintenance of revenue is not currently an impediment to prevention policy. In the early 1970s, however, this was not the case and the Treasury estimates for that time indicated a negative tax elasticity for spirits, i.e. any increase in the tax rate for spirits would have led to a decrease in revenue.

If price elasticities were to remain constant, then governments pursuing a revenue maximisation policy might seek to increase the proportion of tax-in-price to the point when further increases would decrease revenue yields. Once this tax-in-price level has been reached the government should then index the tax rate in order to maintain this ratio. Hence a revenue objective will not necessarily conflict with some policies, such as indexation, advocated by the health lobby.

Price elasticities do not, however, always remain constant and may vary with the level of prices (see Chapter 2 for a fuller explanation of the links between demand relationships and price elasticities). If the elasticity rises sufficiently, then a point may be reached where tax revenues begin to decline with an increase in tax and the authorities may waive indexation until the tax elasticity becomes positive. It is interesting to note that after a period of significant increases in beer taxation, the Treasury has revised its estimate of beer price elasticity from –0.2 to –0.5, suggesting that beer had become more responsive to price after a period of large tax increases. Elasticity of tax revenue is still positive, but fears of increasing price sensitivity and future loss of revenue may partially explain the lack of indexing of alcohol duties in the 1986 and 1987 budgets.

Consideration of the effects of alcohol and tobacco taxation Taxes have effects on consumers and industries, and any adverse effect may act as impediments to health policies based on increasing the tax ratio on alcohol and tobacco.

One aspect of alcohol and tobacco taxation that needs to be considered is whether the taxes are equitable, both across people with different incomes and within groups of people with similar circumstances. The tobacco trade lobby has used the argument that tobacco tax is regressive, that is it falls more heavily on the poor, as a prominent part of their submissions to Chancellors in recent years (London Economics, 1986). Similar arguments have been put forward against the use of alcohol tax (O'Hagan, 1984). The Treasury's own estimates of average tax as a proportion of income do suggest that tobacco and beer taxes are regressive (Central Statistical Office, 1987). Average figures, however, combine both the average levels of expenditure of smokers (drinkers) and the proportion of smokers (drinkers) in each income group.

These issues were examined using data from the Family Expenditure Survey (FES), (Godfrey and Posnett, 1988). Comparisons of the figures for tobacco tax as a proportion of income for 1981 and 1985 over all households would seem to indicate a considerable increase in the burden of tobacco taxes for all income groups. Considering both 'smoking' and 'non-smoking' retired couples together, the average tax as a proportion of income at 2 per cent in 1981 had doubled to 4 per cent in 1985. The figures for 'smoking' retired couples only, however, showed only a small change from 4.4 per cent in 1981 to 5.0 per cent in 1985.

There are fewer problems with equity issues and alcohol taxes partly because the majority of households (over 70 per cent of the 1985 FES) spent something on alcohol during the period of the survey. The proportions of those households with some expenditure do vary across household types, however, with, for example, only 51 per cent of retired households recording expenditure compared to 81 per cent of the non-retired group. If the health argument became more widely publicised and accepted and alcohol consumption changed in a comparable way to tobacco, the distribution of alcohol taxes might become similar to that for tobacco.

There is also a link between alcohol and tobacco taxes which is reflected in the distribution of the joint taxes within income groups. There are considerable differences in the amount paid in tax by consumers who are in the same income groups but have different smoking and drinking behaviour. In 1985, for example, 31.4 per cent of the retired couples in the lowest income group paid no tax on these commodities, whereas nearly a quarter of these households paid an average of £6.55 per week or 12.4 per cent of their disposable income (Godfrey and Posnett, 1988).

Such analyses may indicate that the use of alcohol and tobacco tax as sources of general revenue may have adverse effects. If the objective of taxation is the prevention of social costs, however, governments may be less concerned with the effects of taxes on people with different incomes. The results of Godfrey and Posnett (1988) indicating that smokers pay similar amounts of tax in monetary terms across income groups would not necessarily be considered as a reason for not imposing further tax increases. Similar arguments would also relate to alcohol taxes. Governments may, however, wish to correct any income distribution consequences of taxes by other means as part of other non-health policy objectives. There remain other equity issues, however, such as whether a prevention tax policy for alcohol and tobacco implies that other risky activities, e.g. skiing, motor cycle riding, should be subject to similar taxes (Littlechild and Wiseman, 1984).

Another argument that may be considered is that taxes restrict consumers' choice and affect their welfare by distorting spending patterns. It has been argued that taxing a good for which demand is not very price-responsive does not unduly distort consumer spending patterns. This argument is relevant here because, as reviewed in Chapter 2, both beer and tobacco are generally agreed to have low price elasticities. The estimates for spirits and wine are more varied, but the Treasury's own estimates give price elasticities greater than 1, so that in terms of percentage changes, consumption would fall by more than price increased. These calculations and the rules for the taxation of price inelastic goods are made under a number of assumptions. The analyses have assumed that when considering tax on any one good everything else remains constant. In reality many things may change and these changes may have their own effects on behaviour and revenue that may counteract the calculations made from simpler models.

Examining all the changes that arise from individual tax changes has led some economists to argue that a general sales tax levied at the same rate on a wide range of goods will distort consumer preferences less than varying rates on different goods. The introduction of VAT certainly changed the government's reliance on excise from alcohol and tobacco. VAT accounted for over 50 per cent of the net receipts of customs and excise duties in the financial year 1986/7.

Other rules for optimum taxation have been derived and some analyses, (Kay and Keen, 1985) have suggested that higher levels of taxation on some goods can be justified if the goods are complementary to leisure (a 'good' attracting zero taxes). Clearly alcohol and tobacco goods may be thought to be in such a category.

The level of taxes on alcohol and tobacco goods have effects on industry as described in Chapter 8. Governments may be concerned with levels of employment and effects on the balance of trade arising from tax policy. Also different policies may involve different administrative and compliance costs. At present low administrative costs to the government make alcohol and tobacco taxes an attractive source of revenue. In 1985/6, for example, the cost of collecting VAT as a percentage of revenue duties was 1.04 per cent, compared to 0.69 per cent for alcohol duties and only 0.04 per cent for tobacco. Many of the costs of collective taxes are borne by the industry. If tax policies change these costs may rise and industries may be more unwilling to comply with present tax collection methods.

To summarise, a number of theoretical arguments can be put forward to suggest that governments may find it more difficult to justify alcohol and tobacco taxes as general revenue sources. Governments are, however, likely to maintain revenue at least in the short run and use changes in tax to fulfil macro-economic objectives. In some circumstances revenue objectives policies (such as indexation or high tax to price ratios) may be pursued which also have health benefits, but health and revenue objectives will not always coincide.

Different objectives can lead to different policy targets. So revenue objectives may concentrate on the level of expenditure and the proportion of tax in price, externality objectives focus on price levels, and paternalist policies on the level of consumption. In reality, governments may pursue a mixture of policies. Some of the problems encountered in implementing such potentially conflicting objectives are considered in the next two sections.

POLICIES WITHIN THE PRESENT SYSTEM OF CURRENT TAX BANDS AND BUDGETARY ADJUSTMENTS

Three different types of policy are considered in this section: revalorisation; increasing real rates of taxation; and benchmark policies. All the changes proposed could be implemented without special legislation or a major restructuring of duties. The exact form of the policy would depend on its objective. As the general structure of taxes is assumed to remain the same, it may be expected that the costs of administration and compliance for these taxes will be similar to current rates. As discussed above, the administrative costs are low and governments have shifted many of these costs to manufacturers. Their willingness to bear such costs may, however, be eroded if a health based tax policy is adopted.

Revalorisation

Some degree of revalorisation can be seen as a common component of the revenue and health policies discussed in the first section. As alcohol and tobacco taxes are in part fixed in monetary terms, revalorisation of some form may be needed to maintain revenue. Health groups have been particularly concerned about revalorisation when general prices have risen at a rapid rate. Revalorisation may be seen by health groups as a defensive strategy. For example, in a discussion on tax policy in their document *The Drinking Revolution*, Alcohol Concern state that 'as a first step, the Government must raise taxes in line with inflation' (Alcohol Concern, 1987, p.45).

Revaluing tax rates in line with inflation is the usual but not the only form of revalorisation. Policies could be designed to maintain the value of prices, prices adjusted for income changes, or linked to manufacturers' costs and profits. These policies would have different effects on economic variables such as consumption and revenue. Even if tax rates are maintained at the same level relative to general price levels, the real price of a commodity can change if manufacturers change prices. Technological factors may, for example, lead to lower costs or market changes may lead to the manufacture of a greater proportion of higher quality/price items. Tax as a ratio of price may, therefore, change. Other factors, such as increasing incomes, may contribute to changes in consumption. A policy of revalorising tax rates for increases in general prices, especially over long periods, does not therefore necessarily ensure stable real prices, consumption, or real revenue levels.

Indexing excise tax rates does not necessarily mean equal changes in price for each type of beverage and tobacco. Changes in final price also depend on consequent VAT changes. The effects of a revalorisation policy based on increasing duties in line with general increases in prices are illustrated, with 1986 prices, in Table 3.1.

Table 3.1
Effects of a 5% revalorisation, 1986

Typical good	New price (p)	Change in duty (p)	Net change in revenue, all, £m	Changes in consumption %	RPI change %	RPI change, all %
Pint of beer	71.1	0.9		−0.27	0.07	
Bottle of wine	322.1	4.9	267.4	−1.85	0.03	+0.26
Bottle of spirits	825.1	23.7		−4.16	0.06	
Packet of 20 cigarettes	140.2	2.7		−1.30	0.10	

Source: Godfrey, Hardman and Powell (1986)

As discussed in Chapter 5, indexing rates in line with inflation has been adopted as an official objective of indirect tax policy but, given the present procedures, it is rarely achieved. Some items of government expenditure and tax thresholds have, however, been subject to indexing rules which retain some flexibility. Similar rules for alcohol and tobacco could be devised so that indexation was automatic, unless the Chancellor made explicit proposals for non-indexation in his budget proposals. Such rules would clearly cost the Chancellor some flexibility and may make some other potential health policies more difficult to implement. It would, however, not be costly to administer. The rules would give more certainty for the trade and, therefore, the Government may not be strong opponents of such a scheme. As discussed in Chapter 5, such changes seem acceptable to the public and Parliament. The benefit to health policy is that taxes are maintained in real terms preventing excessive falls in prices.

The major barrier to this policy would seem to be that the actors in the present budget policy making process have considerable incentives to maintain the flexibility and secrecy of annual Budget changes (see Godfrey and Powell, 1985 and Chapter 4). In order to get stronger revalorisation rules onto the policy agenda, pressure from many sources would be needed. Other alterations in the way tax changes are announced may help to ensure regular uprating. Budget changes are often announced in terms of the immediate consequent effect on a typical price and the monthly change in the RPI. Over a full year, however, indexation does not alter overall price changes and the relative price of cigarettes or a pint of beer to other goods will not necessarily be altered by such tax changes.

Indexation of the tax rate to general prices will not automatically fulfil health and revenue objectives. Many health reports have suggested that tax rates should be indexed to incomes as well as to general prices. Alternatively the ratio of tax to price could be maintained. Kay and Keen (1982) suggest that such a policy would not fulfil health objectives. It would be undesirable for the amount of tax per cigarette to fall, if tobacco prices were reduced as costs of manufacturing fell. The value added component of tax for alcohol and tobacco already moves in this way. An alternative means of indexing the tax in price rate would be to revalorise the excise element in line with manufacturers' costs.

A number of countries have adopted price indexing schemes. In Canada different alcohol taxes were linked to changes in average alcohol prices from 1980 to 1984. This system was self-feeding as increases in tax which resulted in increases in price affected the average alcohol price index leading to further increases in tax. Also there were cross industry effects and an increase in the manufacturers' price of beer for example, affected the retail prices of both spirits and wine through the indexing system. Denton and Spencer (1984) examined these effects and alternative indexing schemes, and suggested that the indexing of taxes to a broadly based general price index (such as the RPI in the UK) had a number of advantages.

Increasing real levels of taxation

Many bodies concerned with health would support a gradual increase in the rate of taxation (e.g. Action on Alcohol Abuse, 1986). Implementing a policy of steadily rising tax rates would require a commitment to a health perspective and its consistent application throughout political cycles. Targeting tax policy to real prices as in the quoted example requires a knowledge of manufacturers' costs and profits. As discussed in the revalorisation section, such a policy would be difficult to devise and many have effects on the industry's behaviour.

Table 3.2

Illustrative consumption and revenue changes from various policies

Year	0% yearly real price increase		5% yearly real price increase	
	consumption (lb of tobacco)	annual % change	consumption	annual % change
1985	3.76	–	3.76	–
1986	3.72	−0.99	3.62	−3.65
1987	3.68	−0.99	3.49	−3.65
1988	3.65	−0.99	3.36	−3.65
1989	3.61	−0.99	3.24	−3.65
1990	3.58	−0.99	3.12	−3.65

Year	10% yearly price increases			
	consumption	annual % change	revenue £m (1985)	annual % change
1985	3.76	–	–	–
1986	3.53	−6.13	5609	+6.9
1987	3.31	−6.13	5990	+6.8
1988	3.11	−6.13	6362	+6.2
1989	2.92	−6.13	6743	+6.0
1990	2.74	−6.13	7128	+5.7

Source: Godfrey and Maynard (1987)

Godfrey and Maynard (1987) calculated the effects on tobacco consumption and revenue of policies designed to increase real prices over a five year period using a demand model of the type described in Chapter 2. The projections, based on 1985 data and assuming a 3 per cent growth in real income per annum, are shown in Table 3.2. Using the demand model, consumption in 1990 is predicted to be 5 per cent below 1985 levels even with a constant level of real prices. This fall is due to the effect of the continuing decrease in consumption predicted by the health trend term in the model counteracting the increase in consumption resulting from rising real incomes. A 5 per cent rise in real prices for 5 years is predicted to reduce consumption by 17 per cent and a 10 per cent rise in real prices is predicted to induced a total fall in consumption by 1990 of 27 per cent.

Benchmark policies

Most health policy recommendations have been presented in the form of benchmark targets. So, for example, the Royal College of Psychiatrists suggested that for alcohol '...government taxation policies should be intentionally employed in the interest of health so as to ensure per capita consumption does not increase beyond the present level and is by stages brought back to an agreed lower level' (Royal College of Psychiatrists, 1986). A similar objective has recently been endorsed by the Health Education Authority and all medical colleges (Royal College of Psychiatrists, 1987). The World Health Organisation suggested a reduction of 25 per cent of consumption of both alcohol and tobacco by the year 2000 (WHO, 1984). Finally chancellors have also cited a benchmark of a previous year's tax level when changing tobacco taxes in 1984.

If such strategies are adopted, large changes in taxation can be implied. This is particularly true if some historic price is chosen as the benchmark. So, for example, Godfrey and Powell (1985) and Godfrey, Hardman and Powell (1986) report a number of simulations on tax, price and price related to income to restore values to the mid 1960s or 1970s. Adjusting spirits tax in the 1986 Budget to account for income changes since 1965 would have added over £11 to a bottle of spirits and 33 pence to a packet of cigarettes. Such changes could have large, once for all, effects on the Retail Price Index. Adjusting all alcohol and tobacco duties using 1965 income levels would increase the RPI by over 4 per cent compared to the forecast of 0.2 to 0.3 per cent for simple revalorisation.

Critics of current policy like Alcohol Concern (1987), have suggested that alcohol and/or tobacco should be removed from RPI calculations so that concern about published tax changes would no longer be an impediment to a public health policy. Indeed this procedure has been recently adopted in France. The weights of tobacco and alcohol in the index are, however, not large and therefore only very large changes in the prices of these goods add significantly to the index.

Further constraints on benchmark policies are the existing rules of the EC concerning the relativity of beer and wine taxation. Reflating tax ratios to the 1975 level would result in a ratio of tax on wine to beer of 16.6:1 compared to the present 3.0:1 ratio.

Many effects from such policies can only be estimated with considerable uncertainty because of the unusually large changes in tax they would involve if implemented in any one year. Another way to achieve such objectives would be to phase in changes, as discussed above, but objectives might change during the phasing in period.

ALTERNATIVE TAXATION STRUCTURES

Three policies will be considered in this section. These are: differential taxation; the balance between specific and ad valorem taxes; and the changes in the timing and process of tax changes. There are a number of other alternatives such as direct control of the price of alcohol and tobacco goods. Countries which control the production of these goods by state monopolies already have this option. Such policies would have important implications for industrial competition. These types of policies, or others that may affect price such as the withdrawal of agricultural subsidies, are outside the scope of this chapter.

Timing of tax changes

To some extent the institution of annual budgets makes the adjustment of specific excise duties less of a problem than in countries where such duties can remain unchanged for long periods of time. Another important factor is the inflation rate. With low inflation the minimum gap of a year between revalorisation is less important than when prices are rapidly rising. Even at five per cent inflation, however, this involves an announcement such as 1p or 2p on the price of a pint of beer. A gradual adjustment throughout the year may result in less conspicuous increases and therefore cost less in terms of public support. More frequent tax changes would, however, involve increased administrative costs. Also industry would lose benefits from forestalling tax changes and may suffer increases in cost from, for example, more frequent price notifications to the trade.

Differential taxation

One prevention strategy is to tax commodities on the basis of the harm they create as discussed in an early section of this chapter. Reform of tobacco duties is made difficult because of the harmonised structure of duties across EC countries. For cigarettes, the changes implemented in 1978 switched the tax base from the amount of tobacco they contained to a fixed rate per cigarette with an additional ad valorem component. Changes in the structure of alcohol taxes have already been proposed by Customs and Excise (AAA Review, 1986). These changes relate to the alcoholic strength within types of drink rather than across different drinks. The Government is already constrained by EC rules to tax wines like beer, according to their alcoholic strength, but a similar comparison with spirits has not been made. The Scotch Whisky Association and the Gin Rectifiers and Distillers Association have campaigned for a movement towards taxing all beverages in proportion to the amount of alcohol they contain. There is also support from the health lobby not only for differential taxation, but for restructuring duties to make low alcoholic drinks and mixtures more attractive to consumers. Similarly, the Masham Report (Home Office, 1987) on alcohol and young people recommended increased tax on stronger beers and a rise in tax on cider in line with rates for beer. The concern over alcohol and young people was recognised in the 1988 Budget when some changes in the taxation of beer and mixed drinks were announced.

Existing tax per unit alcohol does vary with the strength of the drink to the disadvantage of low strength drinks (Godfrey and Powell, 1987a). The range for wine was wide within the three tax bands. For example, wine of 14 per cent alcohol content was taxed at 7p per unit alcohol whereas wines of 15 per cent alcohol which fall in the higher tax band were taxed at a rate of 11.3p per unit of pure alcohol. Spirits by contrast are taxed by strength and so excise rates per unit alcohol are equal for all spirits. Prior to October 1988, all beers of lower strength than 3.7 per cent alcohol were taxed at the same rate of tax per pint whatever their strength. The abolition of the minimum duty change of beer, announced in the March 1988 Budget, is intended to encourage both the production and consumption of low alcohol beers. Such calculations refer only to excise rates, the amount of VAT paid in addition varying with the final price.

Two different policies that could be considered are equalising tax per unit of alcohol, or equalising price per unit alcohol and these are also described by Godfrey and Powell. The changes in duty such policies may imply are illustrated by examples applied to 1986 duty rates in Table 3.3. By basing these calculations on beer, the rule of equalising excise per unit alcohol would have resulted in a drop of £2 for a bottle of whisky. If equal price per unit of pure alcohol was the target of policy, substantially different duty rates would have been required, for example, duty on a bottle of spirits would have to be raised by nearly £3.

Another type of policy is to tax more heavily those commodities considered to create the most harm. This may lead to higher taxes on stronger beer as it may be considered that people underestimate its alcohol content. (Historically this is the basis for higher taxes on spirits, although as suggested

Table 3.3

Illustrative changes of tax policies designed to equate tax or price per unit alchohol

a) Equalising excise per unit alcohol at the rate on beer in 1986 plus 3.25% revalorisation

Drink and typical alcoholic strength	Excise per unit alcohol, for typical product, 1986 (p)	Excise change required for policy change (p)
Beer (3.7%)	8.6	+0.6 per pint
Wine (12%)	8.2	+6.0 per bottle
Spirits (40%)	15.7	−206.7 per bottle

b) Equalising price per unit alcohol at the rate on beer in 1986 plus 3.25% revalorisation

Drink and typical alcoholic strength	Price per unit alcohol for typical product, 1986 (p)	Excise changes required for policy change (p)
Beer (3.7%)	35.0	+0.6 per pint
Wine (12%)	22.0	+34.5 per bottle
Spirits (40%)	26.5	+289.1 per bottle

Source: Godfrey and Powell (1987)

earlier there is little evidence that per unit of alcohol spirits cause more harm than other drinks.) This type of policy was directed against high tar cigarettes from 1978 to 1984. The difficulty for this type of policy is to identify correctly the type of alcohol or tobacco good causing excessive harm. It is not clear that the higher rates of taxes on spirits compared to the other drinks can be justified on health grounds.

Whichever type of taxation was adopted, changes in tax bands could have very important implications for producers. Within the present system producers are encouraged to produce goods which minimise the tax on their product. Different tax structures unless carefully constructed may have similar implications. Administrative costs could, moreover, rise steeply if there were numerous tax bands.

Ad valorem versus specific taxation

Ad valorem taxes have the advantage that they will automatically change with price and periodic uprating becomes unnecessary. A change so that all special taxes on alcohol and tobacco were ad valorem in nature may seem advantageous for health policy. Unfortunately, as Kay and Keen (1982) suggest, ad valorem taxes have effects on the structure of the industries. They suggest that ad valorem taxes are useful as a means of controlling excessive differentiation of products whereas specific taxes are more appropriate for revenue raising or health objectives. Specific taxes can be directed as specific characteristics, as described above, and therefore set for a known prevention objective. Ad valorem taxes will only maintain the tax in price ratio and not necessarily constant real prices or constant levels of tax per item. It would also become more difficult, once introduced, to change relative rates of taxation between alcohol and tobacco goods. Within the present system a number of changes in relative rates can be achieved by cumulative changes over a number of budgets, for example, the falling real rate of taxation for spirits.

All the policies discussed in this section would require legislative changes and a consultation process with the industry and other parties. Such negotiations can be costly and policies may be revised during the policy making process. Such policies would require governments to identify their long run aims of a prevention strategy.

EC HARMONISATION PROPOSALS

The changes in the tax system required for a health based policy could be seriously curtailed by the proposal that excise and VAT rates should be harmonised across all EC member states by 1992. The Cockfield proposals, if implemented, would involve large reductions in most of the UK excise tax rates. The proposals as they would effect 1987 rates were given in Parliament and are shown in Table 3.4.

The largest percentage change in duty would be a drop of 88 per cent for table wine. Cigarette duty would also be lower but only by 10 per cent. Calculating the health and consumption effects of such large changes is difficult, but the Government suggests that spirits and wine consumption could rise by as much as a third; beer by 10 per cent; cigarettes and pipe tobacco by 5 per cent; and cigars and handrolling tobacco by about a quarter (House of Commons, 1987, col. 785). An alternative proposal before the EC is from the Europe against Cancer Committee who suggest that tobacco

Table 3.4

Commission proposals for harmonised excise rates

Product		Approximate percentage rate changes
Spirits		−44
Beer		−72
Table Wine		−88
Fortified Wine	15–18% volume	−65
	18–22% volume	−70
Cigarettes		−10
Pipe tobacco		−17
Cigars		−52
Hand rolling tobacco		−55

Source: House of Commons (1987, col.785)

duties should be raised to the highest levels obtaining in the European Community (Powell, 1988).

The proposals have raised considerable controversy in a number of member states. The Prime Minister stated for example '...the Government have fundamental difficulties with the European Community Commission's proposals for the removal of fiscal barriers to trade in the community not least those relating to rates of excise duty on alcoholic beverages and tobacco products' (House of Commons, 1987, col. 733). She also pointed out that fiscal legislation can only be adopted with the unanimous agreement of the member states. Having equal rates for all commodity taxation including VAT would be a serious loss of fiscal sovereignty for all states. Only income and company taxation would be available as policy instruments.

Two separate types of questions are likely to arise in the negotiations over this issue. The first question is whether equal rates of duty are necessary to create an internal EC market. The United States and other federal countries do have differences in commodity taxes between states without internal frontiers. Clearly if taxes are administered as sales taxes, rather than taxes at the manufacturing stage of production, different tax rates may be possible with minimal customs formality. Such a general change in the administration of duties would, however, shift the burden of compliance costs from manufacturers to retailers. Smuggling may also become a more serious problem.

If the member states decide to equalise taxation, the second problem is to decide the form and level of taxation. Clearly, different member states have different industrial pressures and different consumption patterns. Moreover, all will seek to avoid excessive disruption to their home market while maximising their exports to other member states. The wine lobby will be very strong despite its recent decline (Powell, 1989; Chapter 6 of this volume). The UK spirits industry may be keen to open up the European market and welcome lower rates of taxes. In Britain, however, the beer industry is the largest part of the alcohol trade and their ability to trade with member states is hindered by the high transportation costs of their product. Health arguments, other than for tobacco, are not likely to form a large part in these negotiations and therefore the structure of taxation that emerges is unlikely to be in line with health policies. Although negotiations may result in higher overall agreed levels which may improve health outcomes across the community, the UK indicators of harm are likely to be adversely affected. UK tax rates are generally considerably above the average (Powell, 1988) and any compromise is likely to imply a fall in UK excise rates.

The basis for negotiations on the issue of harmonisation remain unclear. The Cockfield proposals were devised by considering the arithmetic average of tax rates and revenue yields over the whole community (Powell, 1988). Kay and Keen (1985) examined some of the possible criteria for a harmonised tax system. In investigating the economic effects of changes in tax structures they concluded that it was necessary for political support to demonstrate that benefits from common levels and structures of taxation outweigh the economic effects of changes. They also suggest ad valorem taxation should be used but only in a limited way with the main part of taxes to be based on product characteristics.

Whatever the final outcome of the EC negotiations, there will be considerable inertia effects. The negotiating process involves a moratorium on tax changes until 1992 and, therefore, it would be difficult to implement any of the policies discussed in the last section. The Chancellor may decide not to uprate taxes annually in order to avoid the possibility of excessive adjustments when agreement is reached. Alcohol taxes are particularly vulnerable to this process.

CONCLUSION

In this chapter, the theoretical basis of alcohol and tobacco taxation, and the effects of implementing a number of alternative tax policies were both examined. From this analysis, it is possible to assess a number of impediments to a preventive health perspective in setting tax levels for alcohol and tobacco. Revenue considerations were seen to be one of the major factors determining government policy. It was, however, shown that although revenue and health objectives may lead to different policy targets, a revenue based policy can also have health benefits. Furthermore, a number of examples of health based tax policies suggest that revenue might increase (at least in the short run) if such policies were adopted.

Revenue yield is by no means the only factor that governments will consider in deciding upon changes in tax rates. Governments will be concerned about adverse effects on consumers and industries, and such concern may be a barrier to the adoption of health based policies. One adverse effect mentioned in the arguments of the trade lobbies is the possible regressive nature of taxation on alcohol and tobacco. The status of such arguments is, however, unclear when health effects are taken into account. The weights given to arguments about equity and liberty will, of course, depend upon the philosophy of the government.

It has been stressed that different tax policies have different implications for the industries. Illustrative changes are provided in Table 3.3 for two types of alcohol tax policy; such changes may lead to substantial differences in relative prices. Some policies, such as automatic revalorisation in line with general prices, may bring some benefits to the trade. The effects of different prevention policies on industries and employment levels will be discussed in detail in Chapters 8 and 10 respectively.

Two important barriers to health based tax policies have been identified. At present chancellors have the ability to vary tax rates in accordance with macro-economic objectives and the need for flexibility impedes the adoption of a more consistent health based policy. The second potential barrier to health policies consists of the EC tax harmonisation proposals. In order to explain further the weight given to such factors and why health policies described in this chapter have not generally been adopted, the present tax policy process is considered in more detail in the following two chapters. Institutional impediments to preventive policy are considered in Chapter 4 and the political and economic factors influencing budget decisions during the years 1974 to 1988 are examined in Chapter 5.

References

Action on Alcohol Abuse, (1986), *Triple A. An Agenda for Action on Alcohol*, Action on Alcohol Abuse, London.

Action on Alcohol Abuse Review, (1986), Differential taxation - is it now on the agenda? *AAA Review*, September/October.

Alcohol Concern, (1987), *The Drinking Revolution*, Alcohol Concern, London.

Atkinson, A.B. and Meade, T.W., (1974), 'Methods and preliminary findings in assessing the economic and health services consequences of smoking with particular reference to lung cancer', *Journal of the Royal Statistical Society*, series A, 137, 297–312.

Berger, D. and Snortum, J., (1985), 'Alcoholic beverage preferences of drinking-driving violators', *Journal of Studies on Alcohol*, 46(3).

Bruun, et al., (1979), *Alcohol Control Policies in Public Health Perspective*, Volume 25, Finnish Foundation of Alcohol Studies, Helsinki.

Central Policy Review Staff, (1979), *Alcohol Policies in the United Kingdom*, Stockholm University, Stockholm.

Central Statistical Office, (1987), 'The effects of taxes and benefits on household income, 1985', *Economic Trends*, 405, 101–117.

Denton, F.T. and Spencer, B.G., (1984), Indexation of Commodity Taxes: A case study of alcohol beverages in Canada, QSEP, Research Report, No. 118, McMaster University, Canada.

Godfrey, C. and Posnett, J., (1988), An Analysis of the Distributional Impact of Taxes on Alcohol and Tobacco, Working Paper, ESRC Addiction Research Centre, University of York.

Godfrey, C., Hardman, G. and Powell, M., (1986), 'Data Note 1, Alcohol and tobacco taxation', *British Journal of Addiction*, 81, 143–149.

Godfrey, C. and Maynard, A., (1987), Price, Consumption of Tobacco and the Economic Effects of a Taxation Policy Designed to Reduce Consumption. Paper presented to the MRC Smoking Research Review Committee, MRC, June, London.

Godfrey, C. and Powell, M., (1985), 'Alcohol and tobacco taxation: barriers to a public health perspective', *Quarterly Journal of Social Affairs*, 1, 329–353.

Godfrey, C. and Powell, M., (1987a), Budget Strategies for Alcohol and Tobacco in 1987 and Beyond, Discussion Paper 22, Centre for Health Economics, University of York.

Godfrey, C. and Powell, M., (1987b), 'Making economic sense of social cost studies of alcohol and tobacco', in *The Cost of Alcohol, Drugs and Tobacco to Society, Papers and Abstracts*, Proceedings of an International Conference published by Institute for Preventative and Social Psychiatry, Erasmus University, Rotterdam.

Harris, J.E., (1980), 'Taxing tar and nicotine', *American Economic Review*, 70(3), 300–311.

Home Office, (1987), Standing Conference on Crime Prevention Working Group, *Young People and Alcohol*, HMSO, London.

House of Commons, (1987), Written Answers to Questions, Parliamentary Debate, 120, No. 27, col. 733.

House of Commons, (1987), Written Answers to Questions, Parliamentary Debates, 120, No. 27, col. 785–788.

Kay, J.A. and Keen, M.J., (1982), The Structure of Tobacco Taxes in the European Community, IFS Report Series, No. 1, Institute for Fiscal Studies, London.

Kay, J.A. and Keen, M.J., (1985), 'Alcohol and tobacco taxes in the European Community: criteria for harmonisation', in Cnossen, S. (ed.), *Tax Coordination in the European Community*, Kluwer Academic, Netherlands.

Leu, R.E., (1983), 'What can economists contribute?', in Grant, M., Plant, M., and Williams, A. (eds.), *Economics and Alcohol*, 13–33, Croom Helm, London.

Leu, R.E. and Schaub, T., (1984), 'Economic aspects of smoking', *Effective Health Care*, 2(3), 111–122.

73

Littlechild, S.C. and Wiseman, J., (1984), 'Principles of public policy relevant to smoking', *Policy Studies*, January, 1–14.

Littlechild, S.C. and Wiseman, J., (1986), 'The political economy of restriction of choice', *Public Choice*, 51, 161–172.

London Economics, (1986), *Who Pays Tobacco Tax?*, London Economics, London.

O'Hagan, J.W., (1983), 'The rationale for special taxes on alcohol: a critique', *British Tax Review*, 370–380.

Perrine, M.W., (1975), 'The Vermont Driving Profile: a psychometric approach to early identification of potential high risk drinking drivers', in Isralstan, S. and Lambert, S. (eds.), *Alcohol, Drugs and Traffic Safety*, Proceedings of the Sixth International Conference on Alcohol, Drugs and Traffic.

Powell, M.J., (1989), *Economic Aspects of Alcohol Policy, Prevention or Profits*, Tavistock, forthcoming.

Powell, M.J., (1988), 'Alcohol and tobacco tax in the European Community', *British Journal of Addiction*, 83, 971–978.

Royal College of Psychiatrists, (1986), *Alcohol our favourite drug*, Tavistock, London.

Royal College of Psychiatrists, (1987), Consensus statement on a Better Response to Alcohol Related Problems prepared at a meeting held on 6th November 1987 at Royal College of Psychiatrists.

Saunders, J.B., (1985), 'The case for controlling alcohol consumption', in Heather, Robinson and Davies (eds.), *The Misuse of Alcohol*, Croom Helm, London.

Wagenaar, A.C., (1984), 'The effects of macro economic conditions on the incidence of motor vehicle accidents', *Accident Analysis and Prevention*, 16, 191–205.

World Health Organisation, (1984), Regional Targets in Support of the Regional Strategy for Health for All, 34th Session of the Regional Committee (EUR/RC34/7) Rev. 1 and (EUR/RC34/13), WHO, Copenhagen.

4 Tax policy: structure and process

LARRY HARRISON AND PHILIP TETHER

In Chapter 3, Godfrey and Harrison showed how manipulating price levels through taxation may be one of the most effective ways in which governments can influence the consumption of alcohol and tobacco. Following Godfrey and Maynard's (1987) calculations, it was predicted that governments could achieve a substantial reduction in tobacco consumption within five years, if it were possible to devise a programme of regular tax increases linked to real prices.

Support for some form of price control has grown, in recent years, with Parliamentary Select Committees, policy analysts and public health campaigners calling for increased taxation on alcoholic drinks and cigarettes in order to reduce consumption and related harm (Expenditure Committee, 1977; CPRS, 1979; Royal College of Physicians, 1983; Royal College of Psychiatrists, 1986). The Government rejected these demands in relation to alcohol, but appeared to concede the argument on tobacco, the Chancellor giving health grounds as one of the reasons for increasing cigarette taxes in the 1984 and 1986 Budgets. Since 1986 the Government has not followed a consistent policy towards tobacco taxation, however, and there is little evidence that future tax decisions will be guided by health criteria. As a senior Treasury official explained to the House of Lords Select Committee on the European Communities, the Government 'takes account' of the impact of economic, fiscal and financial policies on health care, but 'health is unlikely to be the most important consideration for policy makers' (House of Lords, 1985).

It is commonly assumed that governments cannot afford to give a higher priority to public health objectives because they are dependent on revenues from alcohol and tobacco taxes. Large tax increases could lead to a loss of revenue, it is argued, which would conflict with other policy objectives, such as the Government's intention to engineer a shift from direct to indirect taxation. Maximising revenue from indirect or commodity taxation is essential to government plans to reduce income tax rates, and alcohol and tobacco are major sources of indirect tax revenues. Although the tobacco industry's importance as a source of government revenue has declined over the last thirty years, in 1986 it still contributed £5.6 billion in excise duties and Value Added Tax (VAT) to the Exchequer, at current prices. This was approximately 4.1 per cent of all government tax receipts, significantly less than the 12 per cent achieved in 1956, but still a substantial contribution to the Exchequer (Godfrey and Maynard, 1987. Chapter 1 of this volume contains detailed revenue statistics).

Yet the government's income from alcohol and tobacco taxes is not, in itself, a sufficient explanation for the low ranking accorded to health objectives, particularly as excise duties are likely to decline, as a proportion of expenditure taxation, with the growth in revenues from VAT. The Government has increased the rates of VAT and broadened the revenue base since 1979, accentuating the 'fiscal drag' effect of the tax system, whereby every one percent of economic growth produces a disproportionate rise in tax revenue. In a period of economic growth, with rising tax receipts, and with a Government committed to restraining public expenditure, Chancellors are not obliged to maintain revenues from alcohol and tobacco taxation. The tax authorities have already had to adjust to some loss of tobacco revenues over the last thirty years and they could, if necessary, substitute other sources of revenue for alcohol and tobacco taxes.

Important though governments' revenue requirements are, they are not the sole determinant of tax policy. Governments face a number of constraints on policy choice, some of which arise from the nature of the Budget decision making process. While macroeconomic policy is guided by rational planning techniques, such as the use of econometric modelling, the tax system has developed incrementally (Kay and King, 1983). Tax policies are devised and implemented within large public bureaucracies, and it is important to understand how their administrative structures and processes may constitute an impediment to policy innovation.

This chapter examines the structure and process of the UK tax policy system in relation to alcohol and tobacco duties and sets the scene for the detailed analysis of recent budgets in Chapter 5. It is divided into three parts.

The first part outlines alternative theoretical explanations of the policy process. In the second part, the tax policy making process is located within the institutional framework of HM Treasury and HM Customs and Excise, the two departments responsible for advising Treasury ministers on alcohol and tobacco duties. The third part moves from a discussion of administrative structures to the policy process and from discussing the formal constitutional relationship between departments to the informal network of relations between government departments and organisations with an interest in excise duty rates. In conclusion, some features of the tax policy system are identified as obstacles to the use of taxation for public health purposes and ways to counter these impediments are suggested.

THEORETICAL PERSPECTIVES ON THE POLICY PROCESS

Most studies of the British system for determining tax policy have come to the conclusion that it is innately conservative and restricted to incremental change. The present system is not the outcome of rational economic choice. New taxes are introduced in a piecemeal fashion, as either additions to or replacements of existing taxes (Clayton and Houghton, 1973; Kay and King, 1983; Robinson and Sandford, 1983). Within this general incremental framework are three competing theoretical explanations which attempt to analyse why the existing system has been so resistant to change, despite frequent attempts to introduce greater economic rationality to the budgetary process. These explanations include the pluralist model, which stresses the role of government as an neutral arbiter, resolving the competing demands of a wide range of pressure groups; the bureaucratic politics model, which sees policy as the outcome of conflict and bargaining between interests incorporated within the structure of government; and, finally, the administrative constraints model, which explains tax policy as the output of long-established, bureaucratic organisations, which have a massive investment in complicated technical rules and administrative procedures (Hood, 1985). Providing the government machine with a new set of tax regulations and procedures is both difficult and costly, setting important limits on the pace and scale of innovation.

Pluralism   The first of these perspectives, pluralism, is based on Dahl's (1957) critique of studies of the distribution of power in Western democratic societies which claim that power is concentrated in the hands of a ruling elite. Dahl maintains that by analysing a series of concrete historical decisions it can be shown that this hypothesis is false. In the face of opposition from other groups, the policy preferences of the supposed ruling elite are not adopted consistently. Although government may have been oligarchic in the eighteenth century, it is now pluralistic, and power is dispersed widely throughout society (Dahl, 1961). It follows that one of the most significant influences on public policy is likely to be the relationship between government, the electorate and external pressure groups.

The Budget is one area of decision making where winners and losers can be identified, and where individuals and groups have clear preferences for different policy options. It should be possible, therefore, to establish which interest groups have influenced specific Budget decisions by determining which groups attempted to influence decision makers, what their preferences were, and whose views prevailed. In practice, there are a number of problems with this approach. For example, those who benefit from Budget decisions are not necessarily those who exercise power. The benefit could be a 'windfall effect'. As Polsby notes, even if we can show that some groups benefit at the expense of others, 'such a demonstration falls short of showing that these beneficiaries created the status quo, act in any meaningful way to maintain it, or could, in the future, act effectively to deter changes in it' (1980, p.208). Indeed, it may be easier to demonstrate the absence of power than its presence. If, for example, we can show that some groups have consistently failed to benefit from tax changes, we may assume that they have not influenced decision makers. A detailed examination of interest groups and the success or failure of their lobbying activities is contained in Chapter 5; this Chapter is concerned with the extent to which the tax policy making process is either open or closed to external influence or advice.

Bureaucratic politics The bureaucratic politics perspective emphasises the power of senior civil servants to determine policy outcomes and has, as its starting point, a rejection of earlier administrative theories which insisted on a rigid demarcation between policy making and administration. This dichotomy between the business of politics and the business of administration stems from a belief that, in a democracy, politicians should be responsible for policy decisions and administrators for their implementation. Most modern commentators, including prominent Conservative politicians like Bruce-Gardyne and Lawson (1976), regard this as hopelessly naive. It is impossible to make such a hard and fast distinction between policy formation and implementation. Experience gained in implementing policies modifies the original proposals, and it is inevitable that experienced administrators exert an influence on policy decisions.

Those who believe that bureaucrats are political actors, capable of determining policy, either view Whitehall as a 'village' community, functioning on the basis of mutual respect and trust between senior civil servants who are able to form alliances against ministers, or see interdepartmental relations characterised by rivalry and conflict. Many extend the central thesis of pluralism, that power is widely dispersed and not concentrated in the hands of an elite, to include government itself. Far from being homogeneous, government consists of a diverse collection of competing public service bureaucracies, regulatory boards and law enforcement agencies, with little in common apart from their source of funding. On this view, the Ministry of Defence has more in common with its counterparts in other countries than with, for example, the Department of the Environment. Each government department has a different organisational culture or administrative ethos, and each pursues its own objectives, largely in isolation.

The bureaucratic politics model has been developed largely in relation to the analysis of defence and foreign policy, and has not been applied to domestic policy to any great extent (Allison, 1971; Caldwell, 1977; Nossal, 1979). As a hypothesis, it directs attention away from relations between government and interest groups and suggests that tax policy should be studied as the outcome of a political process of bargaining, negotiation and compromise within government. Interest groups often play a part in this process, because departments that lack internal bargaining advantages are forced to seek external support. But civil servants seek alliances with those groups whose demands are in accord with their own objectives; government is not a black box that simply converts pressure group inputs into policy outputs.

The study of bureaucratic politics has been based largely on American evidence, and upon the concepts and methodology of political science. Public choice theory provides a simpler and more rigorous framework for analysing conflict within government, based on an economic model of behaviour. Politicians and bureaucrats are assumed to be rational, value maximising actors who, as Downs (1957, p.2) puts it, 'are significantly— though not solely—motivated by their own self-interests'. Like everyone else, government ministers and civil servants maximise their own utility, and there are 'probably some elements in (their) utility other than the general welfare and interests of the State' (Niskanen, 1979, p.36). Politicians attempt to maximise votes, and enhance their own career prospects, while administrators try to increase their income, status and power, by maximising their departmental budgets.

Civil servants are not certain of ministerial support in their attempts to increase staffing levels and inflate the size of their budgets. Government ministers may fight for their department's expenditure plans within Cabinet, thereby gaining a reputation for being a tough and determined advocate, or they may attempt to reduce public expenditure, winning political support and gaining a reputation for being able to control their own department. The strategy chosen will depend upon its vote-utility and the minister's political support and personal ambition. Like administrators, ministers pursue policies which will maximise their personal utility, and reject those which will not. From a public choice perspective, however, the pursuit of self interest by politicians and administrators will only maximise public welfare in the presence of clear incentives. In order to overcome the resistance the tax authorities have shown to public health considerations, therefore, they would need to be presented with a different set of incentives and sanctions.

Administrative constraints   The administrative constraints model is concerned with the way that reliance on regulations, past precedents and procedural rationality in bureaucratic organisations limits policy choice. The revenue departments are large, impersonal bureaucracies, dealing with mass populations. As there has never been a fundamental revision of the tax system, complicated systems of rules and administrative procedures have evolved over hundreds of years. The tax authorities have a massive investment in the existing structure of regulations and procedures, and change is difficult and costly. Governments have to be able to adapt tax structures to accommodate rapidly changing economic conditions, but, at the same time, believe they cannot afford fundamental restructuring. This is not just because a fundamental revision of the tax system would incur considerable organisational costs, but because of the possible repercussions on international markets and the national economy and the need to maintain a degree of continuity and predictability for tax payers. In such a system, retaining the flexibility of excise duties is of paramount importance, as they enable government to respond rapidly to changing revenue requirements without necessitating a major overhaul of the tax system. As Hood (1985, p.4) notes, enforceability and practicability are the main criteria for selecting or rejecting tax proposals.

    In this Chapter, the three theoretical perspectives outlined above will be used to explain the nature of the tax policy process. Institutional arrangements for determining policy shed light on which model of the policy process has the most explanatory power. The discussion of the decision making process will be preceded by a detailed account of administrative structures.

TAX POLICY MAKING AND THE STRUCTURE OF GOVERNMENT

Probably the first feature of the tax policy system that becomes apparent to the outside observer is its sheer complexity. The second is the political power exercised by the institutions involved. The foremost of these, the Treasury,

80

is the most powerful Whitehall department, exercising a coordinating role in government through the control of public expenditure. The Treasury is well represented within Cabinet. There are four Treasury ministers; the Chancellor of the Exchequer, the Chief Secretary to the Treasury, the Financial Secretary and the Minister of State. Two of the four ministers are Cabinet members, the Chancellor and the Chief Secretary, while the Prime Minister is also First Lord of the Treasury. The Treasury ministers chair many of the key Cabinet Committees, including those concerned with health and social policy, enabling them to influence a wide range of government business. In recent years their influence has been reinforced by the tendency for Prime Ministers to decide major issues outside of Cabinet, in small informal working parties consisting of senior civil servants, the Prime Minister, a few ministers and their political advisers. Treasury ministers have been closely associated with these informal policy making groups, sometimes referred to as the Prime Minister's 'Kitchen Cabinet'.

The two revenue departments, the Inland Revenue and HM Customs and Excise, have direct access to the Chancellor of the Exchequer and are not, as some think, subordinated to the Treasury. Indeed, Chancellors take care not to be identified too closely with the Treasury. According to Robinson and Sandford (1983), the Chancellor avoids sitting on the same side of the table as Treasury representatives in joint meetings between Treasury, Inland Revenue and Customs and Excise officials.

Generally speaking, the revenue departments advise ministers on the more technical aspects of tax administration, while the Treasury is responsible for macroeconomic policy and for advising ministers on the general economic impact of specific taxes, but there is no hard and fast division between policy and administration, or between the work of the Treasury and that of the revenue departments. Like Customs and Excise, the Treasury's Fiscal Policy Group is involved in detailed work on administrative questions, while Customs and Excise are engaged in aspects of policy analysis and are responsible for advising the Chancellor on excise duties.

This duplication of administrative functions seems to have arisen as a result of competition between the departments, with the Treasury moving into areas that were formerly the province of the revenue departments. Until the late 1960s, the Treasury had little experience of revenue collection issues and was not consulted over budgetary matters by the revenue departments, which advised ministers directly. In 1968, Treasury officials decided that they needed to acquire a detailed knowledge of tax collection in order to develop a more 'comprehensive view on tax policy', and they established the unit which, in the course of time, became the Fiscal Policy Group (Robinson and Sandford, 1983). Sections within this Group specialise in policy on direct and indirect taxation, enabling Treasury officials to form their own, independent view of policy proposals.

Because of the overlapping responsibilities between the Treasury and Customs and Excise, both departments are involved in the formation of policy on indirect taxation. However, where individual excise duties are concerned the Treasury takes more of a back seat because Customs and Excise has accumulated greater expertise and has many more people engaged on relevant policy work. In the case of alcohol, for example, Customs and Excise has thirty six administrators working on alcohol policy in one revenue division alone, more than any other department, and ten times the number employed on alcohol policy at the Department of Health.

To supplement the advice received from the Treasury and Customs and Excise, the Chancellor may have special advisers brought in from outside the Civil Service, known as 'irregulars' to Treasury officials. Lord Kaldor was special economic adviser to Chancellors Callaghan, Jenkins and Healey, during the Labour Governments of 1964-70 and 1974-79, and Peter Cropper was political adviser to Chancellor Lawson in 1987. Although the European Select Committees of both Houses of Parliament provide occasional advice or criticism through their review of proposed European legislation, the three main inputs to the decision-making process are the special advisers, the Treasury and Customs and Excise. The Prime Minister's Policy Unit also takes an interest in economic affairs, having been established during the 1974-79 Labour administration largely to provide independent advice on economic policy (Willetts, 1987). Like the Chancellor's advisers, both the Policy Unit and the Prime Minister's special economic advisers tend to be concerned with the Government's macroeconomic strategy, leaving civil servants to provide detailed advice on the specific options for alcohol and tobacco taxation.

The Treasury

In spite of its importance, the department is relatively small, employing about 3300 people. As the Central Policy Review Staff (CPRS) (1979) noted in their report on *Alcohol Policies*, the Treasury has a leading interest in the UK in five alcohol policy areas: fiscal policy, price levels, the balance of payments for trade in alcohol, the economic significance of the alcohol industry and the public expenditure effects of alcohol consumption. The same is true for tobacco. Of these five areas, the Treasury has the greatest involvement in fiscal policy and public expenditure, with almost all of the Treasury's expertise on alcohol and tobacco policy being concentrated in the group dealing with fiscal policy. The Treasury's interest in other areas, like the balance of payments, is extremely general and there are no officials in the relevant divisions with a detailed knowledge of alcohol or tobacco.

The Fiscal Policy Group is divided into two divisions, one dealing with direct taxation and the other with indirect taxation. Alcohol and tobacco duties are the specific responsibility of a branch within the Indirect Taxation Division. The policy responsibility for levels of taxation resides with Customs and Excise, but the Treasury's Indirect Taxation Branch has a general role in advising the Chancellor on indirect taxation, including duties on alcoholic drinks and tobacco. Like Customs and Excise, the Branch is concerned with such things as the impact on government revenues stemming from changes to alcohol and tobacco duties, and there appears to be no clear division between the responsibilities of the two departments.

Most of the Treasury's contacts with other government departments are in connection with their responsibility for controlling public expenditure. The Treasury has experts in its Public Service Sector who monitor the spending departments and enable the Treasury to make an independent assessment of proposed expenditure programmes. The division concerned with monitoring the Department of Health's health expenditure programme, ST2, is in frequent contact with the Department of Health's finance and policy divisions. The Treasury is briefed about the activities of health authorities in relation to smoking and alcohol-related problems and the amount of grant aid being given to non-statutory agencies. It is also informed of trends in smoking and in alcohol consumption and related problems, so that a view can be formed of the implications for future health expenditure.

Unlike Customs and Excise, whose officers are in close touch with the alcohol and tobacco industries because of their responsibility for revenue collection, the Treasury does not have a lot of contact with either industry, apart from the annual submissions on the Budget that trade associations make to Treasury ministers. But senior civil servants from the Treasury and Customs and Excise are frequently required to give evidence on alcohol and tobacco taxation to Parliamentary Select Committees. The European Select Committees contribute to the development of alcohol and tobacco taxation policy through their review of European draft legislation, directives and proposals. Between 1979 and 1986 the European Committees of both the House of Commons and the House of Lords considered European initiatives relating to the consumption and marketing of alcohol and tobacco products on nine separate occasions. Both committees can make policy recommendations, although they tend to be reactive rather than proactive. Their consistent concern is the defence of UK trade interests. They take evidence from a wide range of public bodies and pressure groups and, indeed, they receive evidence from a wider range of witnesses than the departmental select committees. However, when there is a conflict of interests, trade considerations predominate.

Customs and Excise

Customs and Excise is responsible for the collection of VAT, excise and customs duties for the British Government, and agricultural levies for the European Community (EC). As the CPRS (1979) indicated, Customs and Excise has the leading interest in duties on alcoholic drinks, including responsibility for conducting international negotiations. This is also true for tobacco.

Customs and Excise is headed by a Permanent Secretary, responsible to the Chancellor of the Exchequer, with the Minister of State at the Treasury having day to day responsibility for Customs and Excise matters. Policy responsibility for duties on alcoholic drinks rests with two divisions within Customs and Excise headquarters, the Departmental Planning Unit (DPU) and Revenue Duties Division B (RDB), one of two divisions dealing with the technical aspects of excise duties. The other, Revenue Duties Division A (RDA), deals with the non-alcohol excise duties, including tobacco.

The DPU's Policy Branch is responsible for coordinating the Department's contribution to the Budget, covering most indirect taxes, including duties on alcoholic drinks and tobacco. In preparation for the Budget each year, the DPU sets out the future Budgetary options for Treasury ministers, based on their analysis of specific industries and on predictions for revenue yields and elasticities. Alcohol duties may represent up to 20 per cent of their work, tobacco rather less. Other staff in the DPU, particularly in the Statistics Branch, also work on alcohol and tobacco duties. The DPU maintains close contact with the Treasury in the run up to the Budget, and economists at the DPU meet with their opposite numbers at the Treasury to discuss the options for changing specific taxes like beer duty.

Within RDB, the division dealing with alcohol, are six branches, each dealing with a different aspect of taxation. One branch deals with import and export questions. Two branches deal with the warehousing of wines and spirits. One branch deals with the production of wine, spirits and cider, and one with beer. Branch 6 is concerned with the rates and structure of alcohol duties and with work in connection with the Budget. It also deals with international questions, such as European negotiations over harmonising the structure of excise duties. The division is headed by an Assistant Secretary and contains a total of thirty-six staff with responsibility for policy and administration on alcohol duties.

Responsibility for tobacco duties is located in Revenue Duties Division A (RDA), which deals with the non-alcohol duties, but the DPU are also involved, as with alcohol. There are far fewer staff involved in tobacco. Tobacco duties do not pose complex problems of assessment and collection like alcohol duties, which, in the case of beer, are calculated on the Original Gravity of the 'wort', as beer is called prior to fermentation. RDA has only one branch dealing with tobacco, known as RDA1, and as it also has responsibility for hydrocarbon oils it is effectively half of one branch. The branch is headed by a Principal and contains two staff with responsibility for policy and administration on tobacco duties. This includes planning for the Budget and the negotiations over harmonising duties in preparation for the creation of a single European market by 1992.

In addition to the posts in the DPU, the RDB and the RDA, other headquarters divisions deal with accounting and related functions and there is a regional network of Customs and Excise offices. In total Customs and Excise estimate that, excluding administrative services, 1,735 staff were allocated to work on alcohol duties on 31 March 1986; the equivalent figure for tobacco duties was 197. Officers from the local offices work directly with distillers and brewers, assessing duty on the Original Gravity of beer and dealing with warehousing. There are also many people involved in collecting VAT on alcoholic drinks and tobacco.

There is frequent contact, both formal and informal, between the DPU and the Revenue Divisions. There is said to be no need for routine meetings because where necessary, papers are circulated for comment and the DPU receives copies of all Budget briefs. Meetings are held on specific questions when the need arises. Departments with an interest in excise duties—the Department of Health, the Ministry of Agriculture, Fisheries and Food (MAFF) and the Department of Trade and Industry (DTI)—have contact with Customs and Excise over the Budget. The branch of the Department of Health dealing with tobacco is in touch with RDA1 several times a month, one of the links being Customs and Excise's involvement in monitoring the tar content of cigarettes. Because Customs and Excise officials visit tobacco factories regularly, they collect samples of cigarettes on behalf of the Department of Health, which are tested for tar content by the Government Chemist. There is also regular contact between staff in Customs and Excise and in the Enterprise and Deregulation Unit (EDU), a central government task force based in the DTI. All government departments are obliged to liaise with the EDU over their regulatory activities, as part of an attempt to limit the burden placed on business by government regulation.

The most frequent interdepartmental contact is with MAFF. Branch 6 in RDB is in frequent contact with MAFF and both departments provide briefings for each other and copy material to each other. Both departments need each other's advice on technical issues, both are in close contact with the alcohol industry, and both are pursuing similar aims in relation to the

European Community (EC). In negotiations with the EC, both departments favour a package of measures which will benefit the trade and, if possible, open up export markets. Because of the European negotiations, Customs and Excise is also in contact with the Foreign Office. The Foreign Office has officials based in Brussels who coordinate all discussions between HM Government and the EC. Although not usually associated with alcohol or tobacco policy, the Foreign Office has considerable indirect involvement, because it has to be aware of the alcohol and tobacco dimensions in appropriate European negotiations.

While administrators in RDB6 have frequent contact with MAFF over alcohol duties, the Customs and Excise's Tobacco Products Branch (RDA1) does not have a particularly close working relationship with the DTI, the department that has primary responsibility for the tobacco industry. The DTI has never been considered a particularly effective advocate for the tobacco industry. In contrast, Customs and Excise is well informed about the tobacco industry and is able to present the industry's case, at least on revenue-neutral issues like import penetration.

In addition to continual contacts with the alcohol and tobacco industries, both in the course of revenue collection and in relation to the Budget, RDB6 and RDA1 are involved in negotiations within the EC, over proposals to harmonise or approximate the structure of excise duties. The European Commission cannot impose a directive on economic matters, so agreement has to be reached by all member states. Negotiations began in 1972 and have proceeded slowly. There are, on average, only about two meetings each year, because of the detailed technical work that remains to be done and because agreement is proving difficult to achieve. Rates of alcohol and tobacco duty vary widely throughout Europe. If the Commission agreed to harmonise the rates of alcohol and tobacco duties at the highest levels obtaining in the Europe, as proposed for tobacco in the European initiative *Europe Against Cancer*, British duties would actually increase. But the Commission's proposals would result in UK duties being lowered substantially, with a corresponding reduction in alcohol and tobacco prices (European Commission, 1987a; 1987b). The British Government has argued that this is unacceptable because it would have an adverse effect on prevention policy. Both European proposals, one suggesting a substantial increase in cigarette duty levels, the other a reduction of 10 per cent, were being considered by Custom and Excise's Tobacco Products Branch in the Spring of 1988. However, the British Government remained to be convinced that approximating the rates of duties was the best way to remove barriers to trade between member states.

THE TAX POLICY PROCESS

Most commentators have seen the tax policy process as essentially pluralistic (Robinson and Sandford, 1983): power is not in the hands of an elite, it is argued, and the decision making structures are open to influence from a wide range of interests. The introduction of a new tax is characterised by widespread consultation with groups likely to be affected, usually preceded by the publication of a Green Paper setting out tentative proposals. These proposals are frequently modified or even abandoned as a direct consequence of negotiations with interest groups.

The emphasis on pluralism may reflect the fact that much of the literature consists of case studies of attempts at innovation, like VAT, Selective Employment Tax, or some form of wealth tax (Robinson and Sandford, 1983). However, it is important to distinguish between innovation and the annual budgetary process. Where the Budget is concerned, the policy process is characterised by secrecy and the absence of consultation. Government departments and interest groups make 'representations' to the Chancellor each year in anticipation of the Budget, but there is a distinction to be made between 'representation' and 'consultation', the latter implying a greater degree of flexibility and reciprocity. Consultation means that groups are informed of specific tax proposals, and government is willing to enter into negotiations; groups that make representations over a forthcoming Budget can only speculate about the Chancellor's intentions, and they find that there is little scope for bargaining.

In the 1980s, the Government has moved in the direction of greater openness and public debate by publishing public expenditure and revenue figures, together with some indication of the available policy options, in an Autumn Statement in the year preceding the Budget. But the proposals listed for discussion are all at a very general macroeconomic level and there is great resistance within the Treasury to the idea of extending this exercise to the production of a 'Budget Green Paper', or to discussing specific tax changes before a Budget. Apart from the selective use of press leaks to prepare the ground for tax changes, secrecy is always observed when Budgets are being planned because the revenue departments are involved in a complicated strategic game with those who wish to evade or avoid paying taxes. They are faced with skilful, professional opponents, like tax avoidance specialists, who are intent on devising ways to defeat new tax proposals. Many of the short term adjustments to the tax system stem from the strategic manoeuvres and counter-manoeuvres of the tax authorities and their opponents (Hood, 1985).

Before each Budget both ministers and civil servants at the Treasury and Customs and Excise receive representations from the trade associations for the alcohol and tobacco producers, like the Scotch Whisky Association and the Tobacco Advisory Council, and from those involved in the distribution and retailing of cigarettes and alcoholic drinks, like the British Retailers Association. The agricultural side of the alcohol industry, especially those who have been suffering from import penetration like the British hop growers or the cider apple producers, goes through the National Farmers Union. Many of the arguments advanced by these groups are fairly predictable, emphasising the need for tax reductions. According to Joel Barnett, Chief Secretary to the Treasury between 1974 and 1979, the alcohol and tobacco industries are 'politely received but mainly ignored', because they are seen as an 'obviously prejudiced group lobbying in their own interests' (Barnett, 1982). However their profitability and economic circumstances change from year to year and, according to the Customs officials that we talked to, ministers do take note of specific difficulties or new arguments.

Customs and Excise officials tend to receive the attention of these groups rather than their counterparts at the Treasury, because the former have close contacts with the trade over revenue collection issues. The Tobacco Products Branch, RDA1, is in contact with the Tobacco Advisory Council almost weekly over all policy issues, and are informed about problems facing the tobacco industry. The tobacco and alcohol industries thus have a clear advantage, because of this close working relationship, over pressure groups like Action on Alcohol Abuse and Action on Smoking and Health, who also submit their views on alcohol or tobacco duties to Treasury ministers and to Customs and Excise. Most of this activity takes place some months before the Budget is due; documents begin to arrive at Kings' Beam House, the London headquarters of Customs and Excise, in November, after the Chancellor's Autumn Statement but five months before the Budget is announced.

Each year, departments with an interest in the excise duties, like the Department of Health, MAFF and the DTI, are invited to give their views on the forthcoming Budget at a meeting at Kings' Beam House, chaired by a senior Customs and Excise official. There are particularly close working relationships between three of the participants at this meeting: the Treasury, Customs and Excise and MAFF. Until 1988, it was customary for MAFF and the DTI to argue the case for alcoholic drinks and tobacco, while the Department of Health argued the health case. Following the reorganisation of the DTI's responsibilities in January 1988 it is unclear whether they will continue to represent the tobacco industry at such meetings.

Finally, the Chancellor consults the Prime Minister and weighs up the representations he has received from Cabinet colleagues with an interest in excise duties: chiefly the Secretaries of State for Social Services and Trade and Industry, and the Minister for Agriculture. At this point, the process of tax policy formation differs from most other major public policy issues, in that the final decisions are not made in Cabinet with the participation of other Cabinet ministers. The Chancellor merely listens to the views of other ministers, before withdrawing to make his own decisions. Prime Ministers have occasionally overruled the Chancellor on specific issues, as Prime Minister Heath did with Chancellor Barber in 1973, but it is more usual for Chancellors to be left to make the final decision. Prime Minister Thatcher intervened over exchange rate policy in 1988, causing a rift between the Prime Minister's Policy Unit and the Treasury, but this was regarded as exceptional by senior Treasury officials and as interference in the 'Chancellor's prerogative' (*Guardian,* 1988, p.1).

Obviously, Chancellors have to consider whether particular measures might be unpopular with backbench MPs, and both the alcohol and tobacco industries have sizeable lobbies in the House of Commons. Also, public opinion assumes a more important role towards the end of a Parliament; as an election nears, Chancellors are less favourably disposed towards measures that are likely to prove unpopular with large sections of the electorate. But Treasury officials believe that the most important criterion for determining alcohol and tobacco duties is the need for revenue and, although industrial considerations and the effect of proposed tax changes on the Retail Price Index (RPI) are taken into account, it is revenue requirements that determine the structure of the Budget. They argue that chancellors cannot avoid being unpopular with some groups, and the relative strength of pressure groups is less important in tax policy than in most other areas of public policy.

Groups that petition the Chancellor and the Customs and Excise officials each year must believe that they stand a chance of influencing the budget decision, however marginally, otherwise they would not invest so much time in lobbying activities. But most public health campaigners are extremely pessimistic about the prospects of influencing government over tax levels, believing, correctly, that public health considerations do not weigh heavily in the Chancellor's deliberations. Because of the close links which exist between the alcohol and tobacco industries and the tax authorities, who are dependent on each other for information and assistance over revenue collection, access to and influence with government decision makers is not equal and balanced, but skewed in favour of the trade lobby.

On balance, the pluralist model does not provide an adequate explanation of the politics of the Budget. The view of government as a neutral powerbroker, with the most successful groups or coalitions of forces determining policy, does not seem to fit a situation in which groups make 'representations', and there is very little negotiation. Where the Budget is concerned, the Chancellor can be seen as the man in the poker game who knows everyone else's hand. He alone knows all the arguments that will be taken into consideration, and he alone takes the final decision. As Sir Geoffrey Howe observed of his own experience as Chancellor:

> In the end, the economic judgement is that for which the Chancellor is responsible, and one is very conscious of that at the time when it comes to be made. The judgement about the apparently very tough Budget in 1981 was my judgement, and the fact that it is now seen by most people as having laid the foundations for the progress that we've made since then and as an inescapably right judgement gives me more encouragement now than it did in the anxious moments when I was making it. But it really is essentially a personal decision in the context of a welter of advice which one takes from whatever quarter it comes (Young and Sloman, 1984, p.82).

If the relationship between government and external groups is less important in the budgetary process than in other areas of public policy, it is possible that administrators play a correspondingly greater role. Bureaucratic politics can be seen to operate most clearly in relation to the Treasury's attempts to control public expenditure. A minister's reputation with his own senior civil servants often rests on his ability to defend or increase the departmental budget in the face of Treasury opposition. The Rt. Hon. Peter Shore MP, Labour Secretary of State for the Environment between 1976-9, came to believe that there was an adversarial relationship between departments.

> My civil servants behaved as though they were servants of the Secretary of State for the Environment, rather than part of the collectivity of the civil service, and that went just as much for civil servants who had once served in the Treasury as it did for those who had served only in the spending departments. I found throughout my period in office that my civil servants, at any rate, were very pleased indeed when I succeeded in warding off the Treasury. And in providing a whole system of fortification against Treasury assault they were anxious to equip me to fight just as well in the third trench back as I had been fighting in the front line (Young and Sloman, 1984, p.60).

It is clear from the writings and diaries of former Cabinet ministers that government departments do engage in power struggles with each other, struggles that are particularly acute in relation to the distribution of the resources, but which also surface over issues like industrial sponsorship. (See Chapter 7 for a full discussion of departmentalism.) It is, therefore, at least conceivable that civil servants are guided by narrow, sectional interests when advising ministers over tax policy. Thus 'earmarking', which would allocate a proportion of the revenues from excise duties to prevention purposes, would make the Treasury's task more difficult by removing an important area of discretion, and is resisted because it would reduce organisational autonomy. So is indexation, which would link excise duties to the annual rate of inflation, so that they would be automatically adjusted each year in the same way that the threshold for income tax is adjusted. Indexation might also, by simplifying the task of calculating duty levels, reduce the number of staff employed in the relevant divisions at Customs and Excise. Assuming that officials are motivated by the desire to maximise their bureau's budget and size, and improve their own status and conditions of work, we would expect them to find additional reasons why indexation should be rejected.

However, there are reasons for discounting these arguments. The final decision on duty levels rests with Treasury ministers and, according to senior civil servants, the Treasury is the one department that is always under firm political control:

> The knight mandarins of the Treasury are less in charge of the Treasury than any Permanent Secretary is of any other department, because quite frankly, whichever government is elected, it's the ministers in the Treasury who call the shots (Young and Sloman, 1984, p. 115).

Despite the occasional references to broader social and economic objectives in Budget statements, the revenue departments take a narrow view of their function. Their principal task is controlling government income and expenditure and politicians have often accused officials of being immersed in the technical details of the tax system to the detriment of any long term view—indeed, this is one of the reasons that recent governments have introduced independent policy advisers. Perhaps it is not surprising that administrators have strong views on the details of taxation—on issues like the indexation of alcohol and tobacco duties that touch on their central concern with efficient revenue collection. Instead of indexation, which would limit their freedom to change duties in line with revenue requirements, the present administration has favoured a different approach to revalorisation: there is a 'presumption' that excise duties will increase in line with inflation, but the Government can override this when necessary. This form of revalorisation preserves the essential flexibility of the present system of indirect taxation.

The Treasury has similar objections to the 'earmarking' of taxes, which would allocate a proportion of the revenues from excise duties to prevention purposes, in the same way that the Road Fund Licence used to be reserved for expenditure on roads when it was first introduced. The allocation of road fund revenues to the construction and maintenance of roads was abandoned because it led to greater public spending on these items than the Treasury thought warranted. It is precisely because 'earmarking' removes an area of expenditure from the annual round of negotiations over public expenditure that it is resisted by the Treasury. The Treasury believes that 'earmarking' is an inflexible instrument which leads to inefficiency and waste in public expenditure, and this would, of course, conflict with their fundamental objective of expenditure control.

The Treasury's stance on these technical issues gives an insight into its overall philosophy. Whereas public health campaigners see taxation as a potentially useful instrument of social policy, most Treasury officials believe that its sole purpose is to generate revenue, a belief reflected in the department's contribution to the chapter on taxation in the discussion document *Drinking Sensibly* (DHSS, 1981). Their opposition goes beyond the belief that price controls on alcoholic drinks would impose costs on 'those who did not require help', which was the reason given for rejecting controls in the discussion document. They seem reluctant to accept that social objectives have a place in tax policy. According to one of the civil servants we interviewed, 'tax policy is not decided on health grounds, in spite of the Chancellor giving health considerations as one reason for increasing tobacco duties in the 1986 Budget'. From the Treasury's point of view, health is 'just one of a number of competing demands and forms of special pleading'. The Chancellor used the public health argument in 1986 because it was expedient, it was suggested. 'Health considerations' justified tax changes that were really adopted on fiscal policy grounds, and the health arguments were ignored in the subsequent 1987 and 1988 Budgets.

CONCLUSION

Three theoretical perspectives on the tax policy making process are outlined in this Chapter: pluralism, bureaucratic politics and the administrative constraints model. Of the three, pluralism offers the least convincing explanation of decision making. Although the authorities consult a wide range of interests over the introduction of new taxes, the budgetary process is characterised by secrecy. Far from being open and pluralistic, the policy process is designed to discourage participation and is closed to influence from pressure groups. Representations replace consultations, and groups which appear influential may only do so because their demands happen to coincide with government policy objectives. The interaction between group demands and government objectives is complicated as both change over time and a detailed analysis of government-group relations is presented in Chapter 5.

From a bureaucratic politics perspective, tax policy making would be dominated, or at least greatly influenced, by administrators. Where alcohol and tobacco duties are concerned, policy advice is the prerogative of a small number of officials within Customs and Excise and the Treasury. There is no evidence that interdepartmental pressures influence Budget decisions, and although there is an annual exchange of views on the options for alcohol and tobacco duties, there seems to be little scope for bargaining and negotiation. This reflects the unequal distribution of power between government departments. Bargaining between departments, and between administrative units within those departments, takes place in the context of a competition for scarce resources. Departments are more likely to secure or maximise their budgets if they can maintain monopoly control over the market for their service, the provision of policy advice. Where macroeconomic policy is concerned, the Treasury has never enjoyed a monopoly of policy advice. It is in competition with many other agencies, including the Prime Minister's Policy Unit, the Bank of England, and economic advisers to commercial organisations and political parties. But there is less competition in the field of indirect tax policy. Indeed, it has been suggested that the service monopoly established by the Eighteenth Century Excise was the prototype for the modern public bureaucracy (Hood, 1986).

Indirect tax policy is shaped by the practicalities of revenue collection and similar administrative constraints, but the reason that administrative convenience is given such a high priority is that there are few competitive pressures. As Allison (1971, p.81) notes, 'primary responsibility for a narrow set of problems encourages organisational parochialism'. The Treasury and Customs and Excise are able to exercise a high degree of control over the market for policy advice, amounting almost to a duopoly, because of the closed nature of the policy process. The detailed, technical nature of the tax system and the operation of official secrecy restrict discussion of policy issues to a small number of civil servants who control the key resources needed by policy makers: information and expertise. In this way, political choice becomes redefined as technical choice, and power remains in the hands of administrators.

The resistance of Treasury and Customs and Excise officials to many of the policy options outlined in Chapter 3 is a major impediment to the introduction of effective prevention policies. One way to counter such institutional conservatism would be to introduce more competition into the tax policy system so that Treasury ministers would have alternative sources of advice on alcohol and tobacco policy. This could be done within the present administrative structure by appointing an economic adviser to the Chancellor, with special responsibility for developing policies to reduce the social costs of alcohol and tobacco consumption. This would cost little, would stimulate debate within government and would help to ensure that more weight was given to the economic arguments for controlling the price of alcohol and tobacco.

References

Allison, G., (1971), *Essence of Decision*, Little Brown, Boston.

Barnett, J., (1982), *Inside the Treasury*, Andre Deutsch, London.

Bruce-Gardyne, J. and Lawson, N., (1976), *The Power Game: an Examination of Decision-making in Government*, Macmillan, London.

Caldwell, D., (1977), 'Bureaucratic foreign policy making', *American Behavioural Scientist*, 21, 87-110.

Central Policy Review Staff, (1979), *Alcohol Policies*, Reprinted (1982), University of Stockholm, Stockholm.

Clayton, G. and Houghton, R., (1973), 'Reform of the British income tax system' in Robson, W. and Crick, B., (eds.) *Taxation Policy*, Penguin, Harmondsworth.

Dahl, R., (1957), 'The concept of power', *Behavioural Science*, 2.

Dahl, R., (1961), *Who Governs?*, Yale University Press, New Haven,

Department of Health and Social Security (DHSS), (1981), *Drinking Sensibly*, HMSO, London.

Downs, A., (1957), *Inside Bureaucracy*, Little Brown, Boston.

European Commission, (1987a), 'Proposal for a Council Directive on approximation of the rates of excise duty on alcoholic beverages and on the alcohol contained in other products', COM (87) 328/2/ Revision final, European Commission, Brussels.

European Commission, (1987b), 'Proposal for a Council Directive on approximation of taxes on cigarettes', COM (87) 325/2/ Revision final, European Commission, Brussels.

Expenditure Committee, (1977), *Preventive Medicine: First Report from the Expenditure Committee, Social Services and Employment Sub-Committee*, HMSO, London.

Godfrey, C. and Maynard, A., (1987), *Price, Consumption of Tobacco and the Economic Effects of a Taxation Policy Designed to Reduce Consumption*, paper presented to MRC Smoking Research Review Committee, MRC, London.

Guardian, (1988), 15 March, 1.

Hood, C., (1985), 'British tax structure development as administrative adaptation', *Policy Sciences*, 18, 3-31.

Hood, C., (1986), 'Privatising UK tax law enforcement', *Public Administration*, 64, 319-332.

House of Lords, (1985), *Cooperation at community level on health problems*, 13th Report of the Select Committee on the European Communities, Session 1984-5, HMSO, London.

Kay, J. A. and King, M., (1983), *The British Tax System*, Oxford University Press, Oxford.

Niskanen, W., (1979), *Bureaucracy and Representative Government*, Aldine-Atherton, New York.

Nossal, K., (1979), 'Allison through the Ottawa looking glass: bureaucratic politics and foreign policy making in a Parliamentary system', *Canadian Public Administration*, 22, 610-26.

Polsby, N., (1980), *Community Power and Political Theory*, Yale University Press, New Haven.

Robinson, C. and Sandford, A., (1983), *Tax Policy-making in the UK*, Heinemann, London.

Royal College of Physicians, (1983), *Health or Smoking*, Pitman, London.

Royal College of Psychiatrists, (1986), *Alcohol, our Favourite Drug*, Tavistock, London.

Willetts, D., (1987), 'The role of the Prime Minister's Policy Unit', *Public Administration*, 65, 4, 443-454.

Young, H. and Sloman, A., (1984), *But Chancellor: an inquiry into the Treasury*, British Broadcasting Corporation, London.

5 Tax policy and budget decisions

WENDY LEEDHAM AND CHRISTINE GODFREY

The budget process, as discussed in Chapter 4, allows chancellors considerable autonomy in setting the levels of alcohol and tobacco taxes. Chancellors face a number of constraints in deciding tax policy. Conflicting objectives, as described in Chapter 3, have to be reconciled within existing political and administrative barriers to political change. The purpose of this chapter is to examine recent tax changes in order to identify how chancellors decided amongst competing objectives, and what has been the influence of lobby, public and parliamentary opinion.

The time period chosen for these analyses was the years 1974 to 1988. This time span not only involved both Conservative and Labour administrations, but was also a time of changing economic conditions. It is, therefore, a useful period in which to examine potential conflicts between revenue and health objectives in setting alcohol and tobacco taxation levels.

Identifying the different influences on a chancellor's taxation decisions in any year is difficult because of the nature of the decision process, as examined in Chapter 4. Discussions between the trade and health lobbies, government departments and the chancellor are not made public. Statements and campaign material designed to influence public and parliamentary opinion are, however, available. Chancellors may reconsider tax policy if the pressure from lobby groups is reflected in changing public or political opinion. In order to understand how these factors may influence chancellors' decisions on the level of alcohol and tobacco taxation, available material on the actions of health and trade lobbies, and the nature of parliamentary and public opinion are reviewed in successive sections of the Chapter. Chancellors justify tax policy by means of the annual Budget statement to parliament. These statements are examined in the fourth section of the paper, as are alcohol and tobacco tax changes. Finally, some conclusions of the strengths of the impediments to a preventive health-based tax policy identified from the analyses and earlier chapters are discussed.

THE HEALTH AND TRADE LOBBIES

Tax rates on tobacco and alcohol had generally remained at constant levels prior to 1974, as shown in Chapter 1, and neither the trade nor the health lobby were particularly organised around tax policy. But pressure groups were responsive to government policy statements about the health implications of alcohol and tobacco and began to react to the more regular tax changes announced in the budgets after 1974. In this section the activities of both alcohol and tobacco trade lobbies are discussed and their attempts to alter tax policy between 1974 and 1988 are examined.

The tobacco health lobby

The Report of the Royal College of Physicians (1971) had a major influence on public opinion on the link between smoking and health. Other medical organisations and anti-smoking groups became involved in health campaigning and in 1971, Action on Smoking and Health (ASH) was formed to coordinate pressure group activity. The health lobby started to promote the potential use of taxation as an instrument for reducing or alleviating the harm caused by smoking. The argument was taken up by the Select Committee report, *Preventive Medicine*, which recommended that 'an increase in duty to achieve price increases sufficient to reduce public consumption should be imposed annually' (Parliamentary Expenditure Committee, 1977). The ASH campaign recognised that public support was important in persuading the Chancellor to adopt such policies and campaigns during this period focused on influencing public opinion.

During the next two Conservative administrations however, the health lobby attempted to adapt their arguments on taxation to new Conservative policies. The stated government policy of switching from direct to indirect taxes prompted the health lobby to put pressure on Treasury ministers to increase tobacco duty levels. In their arguments, they stressed the social and economic costs to the community of smoking.

As well as submissions to chancellors, the health lobby tried to win the support of key influential groups and professions. Brian Bailey, the Chair of the Health Education Council (HEC), wrote to all Regional Health Authorities, asking them to petition the Chancellor to increase duty rates and also to encourage similar action by the health authorities in their regions. The HEC's aim was to get the organisations primarily responsible for health care to focus on prevention policies and to ensure that the Chancellor was aware of the national and local medical support for a health dimension in budgetary policy. ASH also continued to try to gain support from the party in power by lobbying groups within it, such as the Conservative Women's National Committee and the Tory Reform Group.

Increasingly sophisticated campaigns continued after the 1983 election and the appointment of Nigel Lawson as Chancellor. The health lobbies widened their activities. ASH provided material to support parliamentary groups, such as the All Party Group for Action on Smoking and Health, in debates. They also strove to meet Treasury ministers personally as well as giving written submissions. The health lobbies were thus able to make calculated demands that would fit more closely with the Chancellor's anticipated budget strategies. For example, ASH became aware from meeting Customs and Excise officials that the Chancellor's policy was to raise duties in line with inflation. To campaign for such increases was, therefore, not productive and they changed their campaigns to demand price increases in excess of the inflation rate. The British Medical Association (BMA) had also increased its anti-smoking activities and in mid 1987, ASH and the BMA co-operated in order to form a more long term policy of campaigning for large tax increases.

The tobacco trade

From 1976, the tobacco trade became increasingly concerned about the effects of changing tax structures (see Chapter 1 for details) and the effects of health information. By 1978, cigarette sales had begun to decline and the industry had failed to increase exports sufficiently to prevent some drop in production. The industry had reduced its labour force and there had been a loss of 1,200 manufacturing jobs between 1977 and 1978 (see Chapter 8 for the reasons for these job losses). The Tobacco Advisory Council, the trade association of the UK tobacco manufacturers, reacted to these pressures by making written annual submissions to the Chancellor. The trade lobby, as part of its campaigning activities, refined its arguments against taxation to focus not simply on the effects on sales, but on more highly political issues, such as the effects on employment, particularly in the regions. Further arguments against tax increases were produced. The trade lobby argued that since tax duties already represent 74 per cent of the price of cigarettes, further increases in tax rates would be likely to lead to falls in revenue. Moreover, it was suggested that tax increases would set off an inflationary spiral. The trade lobby highlighted the UK tax rates relative to other EC countries, pointing out the threat of cheap imported cigarettes to the UK industry and the resulting employment consequences.

Under a Conservative Chancellor after 1979, the trade lobby developed campaigns to win over public support, as well as increasing their private, direct lobbying of officials in the budget making process. Particularly after 1981, when tobacco taxation was increased twice, public opinion campaigns, such as the nationwide smokers' petition, were initiated. Considerable sums in pre-budget advertising began to be spent regularly, for example £629,000 in 1982 (*The Times,* 1982) and £250,000 in 1983 (*Sunday Times,* 1983).

In 1986, the tobacco industry's tactics were reviewed. Closer links were forged with tobacco retailers and their association, the Tobacco Alliance. A more aggressive stance of a total freeze on tobacco taxation was adopted and MPs rather than the public were the main target for the campaign. Following this campaign, a group of Labour MPs lobbied the Chancellor about the growth of cheap foreign imports.

The tobacco trade and health lobbies have both developed their arguments taking into account the political philosophies of the party in power. As the period progressed, both lobbies recognised their ability to influence directly the Chancellors' budget decisions, and have therefore widened their lobbying activities. The tobacco trade has engaged in direct lobbying of parliament and spent considerable sums attempting to influence public opinion with a strategy of introducing a growing number of impediments to increased tobacco taxation. The health lobby also widened its activities and sought to gain acceptance that tobacco taxation should be fixed in line with health objectives.

The alcohol health lobby

The alcohol health lobby has faced more difficulties than the corresponding tobacco groups. In 1974, the relationship between alcohol and the consequences for health was not widely accepted. However, rapidly rising levels of consumption and indicators of harm during the 1970s did begin to change and influence medical opinion. This was recognised in the 1977 Select Committee report *Preventive Medicine*, which recommended that the Government maintain the price of alcohol relative to average incomes. The Government demonstrated a strong reluctance to take this position in the White Paper, *Prevention and Health* (1977), and later in the suppression of the Central Policy Review Staff Report (1979) which contained similar recommendations. However, some recognition of the potential of taxation as a control policy was given in the DHSS document *Drinking Sensibly* in 1981. This report rejected systematic use of tax policy, but stated that health and social implications would be 'take(n) into account when changes in duty and wider taxation policy are considered' (DHSS, 1981).

The pressure groups Alcohol Concern and Action on Alcohol Abuse (AAA) were formed in the early 1980s. Like ASH, these groups have not only petitioned government about tax and other control policies, generally, but have met Treasury ministers to discuss their pre-budget submissions in direct lobbying. They have sought to increase public awareness of tax policy by educational campaigns and by publicly condemning the Chancellor's failures to increase alcohol duties in the 1986 and 1987 budgets. These groups face considerable difficulties in changing public opinion, given the high proportion who drink and the unclear health arguments on the relationship between moderate drinking and adverse health effects.

There has been some variation in the demands of alcohol lobbies on the Chancellor possibly because the outcomes of different tax policy options are uncertain. For example, Alcohol Concern have argued that 'stabilisation is the best that can be hoped for from taxation policies' (Alcohol Concern, 1987, p.36). On the other hand, AAA state that one of their objectives must be 'to reduce per capita consumption by 30–45 per cent over the next six years by means of appropriate changes in rates of taxation' (AAA, 1986, p.5). More recently, however, there has been some attempt to co-ordinate policy objectives by the health lobby. A meeting of the Medical Colleges, AAA, Alcohol Concern and the Health Education Authority stated that 'we would recommend that Government fiscal policy should be initially employed to ensure that per capita consumption is gradually reduced' (Medical Colleges, 1987).

The alcohol trade

Certain issues such as policies to equalise tax by alcohol content, as discussed in Chapter 3, have been promoted not only by the health lobby but also by some of the trade groups. Lower strength beverages are discriminated against by the present tax bands, and the Scotch Whisky Association in their submissions to the Chancellor express the view that drinks should be taxed according to their alcoholic content. Because of the possibility that consumers may substitute different drinks as prices vary, different sectors of the alcohol industry have competing interests and there is a long history of different parts of the industry campaigning against one another (Weir, 1984). The different tax structures for different alcoholic beverages mean that there is not a single industry wide perspective on appropriate tax levels, and the alcohol trade and health lobby occasionally find themselves making the same demands on the Chancellor. In 1982, for example, the Licensed House Managers and Tenants joined forces with the National Council on Alcoholism to press the Chancellor to impose excise duty on home-made liquor.

Unlike tobacco, the alcohol trade lobby has been less concerned about highlighting the impediments to the policies suggested by the health lobby. Trade submissions to the Chancellor have tended to be claims for special status and demands for specific actions to facilitate the development of the industry. The brewers for example have considered themselves to be discriminated against by the levels of duty imposed compared to other alcoholic drinks (Brewers Society, 1986). The Scotch whisky industry has continually pressed for the introduction of an allowance to take account of the inflationary factor on maturing stocks of whisky, in order to reduce discrimination in the present tax system.

The complexities of the alcohol trade and the relatively uncoordinated approaches of the health lobby have resulted in disparate demands on the Chancellor. The trade tends to pursue sectional interests in lobbying government and parliament on taxation issues. There has also been little evidence of an effective joint approach by the health lobby.

PARLIAMENTARY SUPPORT FOR A PUBLIC HEALTH PERSPECTIVE

Both the alcohol and tobacco industries engage in considerable lobby activity to manipulate tax policy. Their direct impact on the budget policy process is unclear, but they have also sought to mobilise parliamentary opinion in their interests. It is clear that parliamentary opinion can significantly influence budget decisions during the period between the budget announcement and the Finance Bill. For example, on two occasions, in 1977 and 1981, parliamentary opinion has forced the Chancellor to withdraw a petrol duty increase announced in the budget, and the revenue shortfall in 1981 was made up using tobacco duties. As well as directly influencing budget decisions, parliamentary opinion can set limits on the acceptability of chosen tax levels. The channels through which backbench MPs can express their opinions in Parliament, outside debating legislation, are Parliamentary Questions, Adjournment Debates, and Early Day Motions. In Parliament, members may be speaking in either a personal capacity, as a party member, as a constituency representative or on behalf of a sponsoring organisation.

Parliamentary questions are directed at the ministers of each department. They may be tabled by MPs as often as they wish, but are frequently used to try to draw ministers' attention to the issue in question. Parliamentary questions relating to alcohol and tobacco taxes between 1974 and 1987 were analysed and allocated to the following categories.

Table 5.1

Types of parliamentary questions 1974 to 1987

Alcohol and tobacco trade	61
Taxes' role in the economy	32
Health and welfare implications	21
Constituency interests	9
Consumer interests	7
Other	14

Source: House of Commons, *Parliamentary Debates,* 1974 to 1987.

These details show that there were almost twice as many questions relating to the alcohol and tobacco trade as the next largest category, the role of alcohol and tobacco taxes in the economy. Questions relating to the economic role of alcohol and tobacco would be of interest to opposition and government MPs as a way of attacking or defending government policy, and so might be expected to form a significant proportion of the whole. The ratio of questions in these two categories points to the dominance of trade interests in Parliament, particularly the alcohol industry.

The content of the questions in the trade category was examined to assess why the alcohol and tobacco industries made such extensive use of parliamentary channels. There have been several questions about issues concerning these industries which require continuous pressure in the long term to effect change. The major issues occurring over the 13 year period have been duty deferment and the method of collecting taxation for HM Customs and Excise; levels of duty increases; and the implications of EC harmonisation proposals. These issues are also addressed in the trades' annual pre-budget submissions to the chancellor, indicating the trades' perceived need to maintain a permanent relationship with government outside their sponsoring departments (see Chapter 7), as well as a channel for short term strategies in response to issues of immediate concern.

Parliamentary questions relating to the role of alcohol and tobacco taxes in the economy indicate the role that parliament plays in monitoring budget policy and the general parliamentary recognition of the distinctive revenue raising abilities of these goods. When budget policy fails to meet its financial objectives, more of these types of questions are tabled. For example, in 1983, when there was a shortfall on revenue estimates from alcohol and tobacco duties, the matter was raised in a number of parliamentary questions.

The health and welfare issues addressed in parliamentary questions do not necessarily reflect the importance attached to parliamentary channels by the health lobby, especially regarding alcohol. Parliamentary questions are directed at a particular government department and raising health issues with Treasury ministers severely limits the type of answer requested. Between 1975 and 1980, however, there were a number of questions concerning the re-distribution of alcohol and tobacco duty revenue to the health and social services. This was the period of the first big public expenditure cuts and the parliamentary questions were probably aimed at making party political points about general economic policy, rather than a direct concern for prevention policy. After 1980, parliamentary questions in this category were more directly related to a prevention policy, although the numbers concerned were small. The system of parliamentary questions has not been a particularly useful channel for the health lobby in its efforts to promote the use of tax increases to control consumption.

Taxation as a strand in prevention policy has been given a higher profile in Adjournment Debates. Three out of the four debates relating to alcohol and tobacco taxation that took place between 1974 and 1987 urged the use of fiscal policy to reduce consumption. The debates were all initiated by Conservative MPs with interests in alcohol and tobacco problems.

The health effects of consumption were discussed in the debates, as was the Government's dependence on revenue, but responses from ministers were non-committal. Comments in these debates illustrate the departmentalism that acts as a barrier to developing a health perspective to tax policy in government. In one debate, a Health Minister stated that it was not his place to comment on fiscal policy. (See Chapter 4 for a discussion of departmental relationships in tax policy.) In a further debate about the possibilities of removing alcohol and tobacco from the Retail Price Index (RPI), a Treasury minister argued that the health consequences of taxation policy were not really a matter for the Treasury.

Adjournment Debates provide a platform for MPs with a personal interest to urge a re-thinking of policy. However, the small chances of winning the ballot for a debate and the pressure to address more immediate issues makes this channel a very weak and haphazard expression of parliamentary opinion. Early Day Motions are probably the best indicators of backbench opinion because they do not have to address government departments and they indicate the number of MPs supporting the motion. Of the eight tabled between 1974 and 1987 relating to alcohol and tobacco taxation, seven urged the Chancellor not to increase duty on these goods. However, the Motions were not well supported with an average of only eight signatures. It is difficult to determine the motivation behind tabling these motions, but consumer and constituency interests were possibly the main influences. Early Day Motions do not reveal significant numbers of backbench MPs with strong opposition to the use of tax policy in the prevention of tobacco and alcohol related harm.

PUBLIC OPINIONS ABOUT TAXING ALCOHOL AND TOBACCO

The relatively low priority given to the health consequences of tax policy by most backbench MPs may be an indication of the lack of popular acceptance of the legitimacy of such control policies. The relationship between public attitudes, behaviour and policy is complicated and depends very much on the nature of the issue (Leigh, 1976). With budget policy, negative public attitudes may not necessarily be as constraining as with other issues. Mass public opinion on alcohol and tobacco tax policy must be understood not just in the context of widespread public disapproval of taxation in general, but of an understanding that duty rates are subject to annual review and that losses from higher duty rates may be compensated for by other tax measures.

Although the nature of public opinion data makes it very difficult to identify trends over time, there have clearly been more developments with tobacco than alcohol. Tax hikes on tobacco have accompanied a growing acceptance of the arguments about smoking and health and a fall in the number of people smoking (see Table 1.6, Chapter 1), without the government losing a substantial amount of public support. However, the public opinion data indicate that this public acceptance has a ceiling. Table 5.2 shows public opinion data from various sources over time. Generally, there is a greater percentage of respondents indicating approval of increased taxation on cigarettes. In 1981, however, the poll showed a greater percentage disapproving of increased taxation. Prior to 1981, price increases of between 3p and 7p following the budget had become the norm. The 1981 April budget added 14p to the price of cigarettes and, later in the year, a further duty of 3p was added.

Public acceptance of high tax levels may also be a result of what appears to be a cynical attitude towards government using tax policy for health objectives. In Marsh and Matheson's (1983) survey, 68 per cent of smokers and 65 per cent of ex-smokers agreed with the statement that the government was too dependent on tobacco tax revenue to discourage smokers.

Table 5.2
Approval/disapproval of increased taxation on cigarettes

Date	Approve %	Disapprove %	Indifferent %	Don't know %	Base	Source
Apr 1975	51	36	–	13	N/K	1
Aug 1975	48	45	–	7	N/K	1
Oct 1987	41	38	17	–	3938	2
Feb 1976	53	40	–	7	N/K	1
Apr 1976	42	37	18	–	4023	2
Apr 1977	46	45	–	10	N/K	1
Nov 1980	52	37	–	12	1024	1
Dec 1981	36	42	19	–	3899	2
Dec 1982	45	38	14	–	3671	2
Dec 1984	41	34	22	–	3748	2
Dec 1985	43	33	22	–	3330	2
Dec 1986	48	30	21	–	5398	2

Sources: The Gallup political index

Survey by National Opinion Polls, extracted from DHSS records.

There is less information available about public attitudes to alcohol taxation (Leedham, 1987). Policy makers do not have high expectations of wide public acceptance of increasing tax levels on alcohol. Consequently surveys tend to address the issue of whether existing control policies are still appropriate, rather than considering alternatives. In surveys that do suggest alternative policy options, there seems little support for high levels of taxation. A study for the Health Education Council (Wood, 1986) reveals that 73 per cent of respondents thought that it was a bad idea to increase tax on beer in order to cut down the amount people drank, with a corresponding figure of 70 per cent for spirits. Almost all those who thought it was a bad idea said that it would not have the intended effect. These beliefs were highly correlated with the amounts people said they drank.

Public opinion data indicate a public awareness of the importance of the revenue raising ability of alcohol and tobacco duties, and acceptance of high levels of taxation may be more related to stoical attitudes to tax burdens than to a belief that tax hikes would reduce consumption.

Chancellors' budget statements and decisions on alcohol and tobacco taxation can be examined in order to obtain some evidence on the influence of the health and trade lobbies which were discussed above. There are, of course, many other influences such as consideration of general revenue and economic management (see Chapter 3). The importance of the different influences may be indicated by the arguments used to justify tax changes. In the period 1974 to 1988, there were three chancellors and their budget statements are now considered in turn.

Denis Healey, 1974 — 1979

Table 5.3

Annual changes in excise tax rates and retail prices, 1974–78, (%)

Year of budget	RPI (March to March)	Beer	Wines[a]	Spirits	Cider	Cigarettes[b]
1974	13.5	29.3	56.6	10.0	-	34.5
1975	17.5	46.1	95.2	29.9	–	33.3
1976	21.1	15.8	10.5	11.5	–	0.8
1977	16.7	10.0	10.0	10.0	10.0	23.2
1978	9.1	0.0	0.0	0.0	0.0	0.0

a. Prior to 1 January 1976, wine duty refers to basic duty per gallon at the lower rate. From 1976 it refers to the lower wine duty for wines less than 15 per cent alcohol.

b. As cigarettes are subject to more than one duty, the specific tax rate (including the special and ad valorem duty but not VAT) was calculated for a typical product. For other commodities changes in duty were calculated from basic duty rates.

Sources: RPI figures from Department of Employment, *Employment Gazette,* London, HMSO, (monthly).
Excise rates from Annual Reports of the Commissioners of Her Majesty's Customs and Excise, London, HMSO, various years.

As can be seen in Table 5.3, there were frequent budget changes in alcohol and tobacco taxes during this period. The frequency of changes introduced by Mr Healey was in contrast to earlier years (see Chapter 1). It is difficult to see any relationship with changes in general prices, or any other pattern in the excise rates presented in Table 5.3. The effect of excise tax changes on the final price of alcohol and tobacco goods depends on the additional amount of VAT implied by these tax changes. In Table 5.4, it can be seen that the percentage changes in price and the proportion of tax in price have varied both over the period and between different goods. The effects on beer prices, for example, varied from 0 to 10 per cent, but were lower than those for whisky and cigarettes.

Table 5.4

Changes in the prices and tax incidence for typical products as a result of budgets, 1974–78

Year of budget	Beer (pint)	Whisky (bottle)	Cigarettes (20)
a) Change in typical price (%)[a]			
1974	6	7	16
1975	10	17	17
1976	4	7	8
1977[c]	3	6	15
1978	0	0	0
b) Duty and VAT as % price[b]			
1974	32.4	90.1	70.0
1975	35.7	85.5	69.3
1976	33.5	82.0	69.6
1977[c]	32.3	80.1	63.8
1978	30.5	78.4	70.2

a.   These figures are calculated from the estimated change in price of a typical product announced in the Budget as a percentage of the post budget price.

b.   These figures are calculated from total excise and VAT as a percentage of the post budget price.

c.   These changes reflect the use of the regulator in the autumn of 1976. The 10 per cent increases in duty levels were consolidated in the 1977 Budget.

Sources: Budget statements and annual reports of the Commissioners of Her Majesty's Customs and Excise, London, HMSO.

It is necessary to consider the economic, revenue, political and health objectives of the Chancellor as expressed in budget statements to determine the reasons for the pattern of tax changes. Most emphasis in such statements is given to broad economic objectives. The period from 1974 has been a time of difficult economic conditions. The two oil crises in the 1970s, high inflation and, later in the period, high levels of unemployment contrast with the period prior to 1974 when management of the economy had consisted of fine-tuning with relatively low levels of inflation and unemployment. All three chancellors were concerned with the level of the Public Sector Borrowing Requirement (PSBR), i.e. the difference between government expenditure and revenue. Being an important source of revenue (see Chapter 1), taxes on alcohol and tobacco became more closely linked to the management of the economy. The use of alcohol and tobacco taxes for such purposes was clearly illustrated in 1976. Following a sterling crisis, the Chancellor applied for support from the International Monetary Fund (IMF) and the subsequent agreement set limits to domestic credit expansion. In order to reduce the PSBR, the regulator was used to increase alcohol and tobacco by 10 per cent in the autumn mini-budget. (The regulator is a procedure by which chancellors can increase excise duties between budgets without a change in legislation.) The action shows the importance to chancellors of maintaining flexibility in raising revenue and the potential use of alcohol and tobacco duties in periods of economic uncertainty or crisis, (for further discussion see Godfrey and Powell, 1985.)

The Chancellor did, however, describe a number of constraints on his ability to raise revenue from alcohol and tobacco duties during his period of office. One of the factors he considered was the effect of inflation. As indicated by the figures of Table 5.3, large changes in the real value of excise duties can occur during periods of rapidly rising prices. The Chancellor recognised the need to revalorise duties, and statements expressing this need became a frequent feature of his and the succeeding chancellors' speeches. Announced tax changes which are seen to add directly to increases in the RPI are difficult to implement in periods when inflation is of major political and public concern. Additionally, in 1974 the Chancellor's ability to raise taxes was constrained by the previous Government's pay agreement. Pay awards were linked to the general movement of prices. A change in the RPI could trigger the thresholds built into the agreement and reinforce the inflationary spiral. This example illustrates how other policies can impinge on the freedom to pursue specific alcohol and tobacco tax objectives.

Another limiting factor on changes in alcohol and tobacco taxes identified by the Chancellor was the effect of taxes on people with different incomes. To justify expenditure taxes which normally fall more heavily on the poor than the rich, the Chancellor introduced in his 1974 Budget the notion of essential and less essential goods (House of Commons, 1974, col. 308). It is clear that wines, spirits and tobacco were seen as less essential goods. The Chancellor's position on beer was more ambiguous and he stated 'in normal circumstances I should have preferred not to change the duty on beer' (House of Commons, 1974, col. 310). During this period of office, the Chancellor generally imposed lower increases on excise rates for beer than other alcoholic drinks. In 1976 the Chancellor also suggested that tobacco increases were also limited by distributional concerns. He stated: 'However, I had to pay some regard to the level of prices and to the burden on those, particularly the poor, who find it difficult to cut back on their smoking' (House of Commons, 1976, col. 260).

There was little evidence in any budget statement that either the health or the trade lobby affected the Chancellor's decisions. There was, however, some evidence that there was some change in attitude over the period to the use of tobacco tax to achieve health objectives. In 1974 the Chancellor stated '... I do not necessarily subscribe to the principle that the consumption of tobacco products should be cured by fiscal means' (House of Commons, 1974, col. 311). In the 1976 Budget, however, he expressed the view that there was 'a strong case on health grounds as well as revenue grounds for increases in the taxation of tobacco' (House of Commons, 1976, col. 259). Further, in 1978, the Chancellor introduced a tax on higher tar cigarettes specifically to alter consumption habits. There was, however, no parallel concern announced for the health consequences of alcohol consumption.

Another feature of Table 5.3 is the lack of changes in duties in the pre-election budget of 1978. Increases in cigarette and beer prices may be thought to be unpopular with the electorate.

Geoffrey Howe, 1979 – 1983

The basis of the incoming Conservative government's economic policy was stated in the first budget of the administration. The major aims of controlling the money supply (through the PSBR) and shifting the burden of taxation from direct to indirect taxes had implications for excise duties on alcohol and tobacco goods. Such policy aims suggest that alcohol and tobacco goods could be taxed more heavily. The effects of budget changes on excise rates and prices are given in Tables 5.5 and 5.6. It can be seen that excise rates, particularly for beer and tobacco, were substantially increased over the period.

In his first budget, the Chancellor used an increase of the VAT rate from 8 to 15 per cent both to raise additional revenue and to shift the balance from direct to indirect taxes. Excise rates were not changed, but the increase in VAT did substantially affect alcohol and tobacco prices as can be seen in Table 5.4. In 1980 and subsequent years indirect taxes were increased and the Chancellor, when announcing changes, seems to have been mainly concerned with revenue yield. In 1981, for example, he stated: 'I am proposing to increase the excise duties to produce in total about twice as much additional revenue as would be required to compensate for one year's inflation', (House of Commons, 1981, col. 773). A policy based on revenue

Table 5.5

Annual changes in excise tax rates and retail prices, 1979–1983, (%)

Year of budget	RPI (March to March)	Beer	Wines	Spirits	Cider	Cigarettes
1979	9.8 (14.5)[a]	0.0	0.0	0.0	0.0	1.7
1980	19.8	22.5	13.8	13.7	13.7	19.9
1981	12.6	37.9	16.9	14.6	19.0	31.1
1982	10.4	13.3	12.2	6.4	13.3	13.8
1983	4.6	5.9	5.8	5.0	18.8	5.4

a. Figure in brackets refers to the March 1978 to June 1979 changes. The Budget was presented in June.

b. See Table 5.3 for definition of terms.

Sources: See Table 5.3.

Table 5.6

Changes in the prices and tax incidence for typical products as a result of budgets, 1979–83

Year of budget	Beer (pint)	Beer (bottle)	Whisky (bottle)	Wine (20)	Cigarettes
a) Change in typical price (%)					
1979[a]		5	5	6	9
1980		5	8	4	7
1981		8	8	6	15[b]
1982		4	4	4	5
1983		2	3	2	3
b) Duty and VAT as % price					
1979		32.3	78.2	39.4	69.7
1980		33.6	77.8	41.6	70.7
1981		37.8	77.8	44.0	73.7[b]
1982		38.1	76.9	45.6	74.6
1983		37.9	76.8	45.3	73.8

a. Although the excise rates were unchanged for alcoholic goods, VAT was raised from 8 to 15 per cent.

b. Extra duty of 3.5p per packet was imposed on 8.7.81, this was equivalent to 4 per cent of the new price of a packet of cigarettes.

For details of the calculations see Table 5.4.

Sources: See Table 5.4.

objectives does not require that duties on all goods are raised equally and Geoffrey Howe increased the duties on beer and tobacco proportionately more than those on wines and spirits.

The flexibility of indirect taxation in accommodating shortfalls in revenue was demonstrated in 1981. The Government dropped a proposal to increase derv duty in the face of strong opposition and the Chancellor was able to increase tobacco taxes to make up the resulting projected loss of revenue.

The Chancellor stated in the 1982 Budget that 'for the Excise duties there has grown up in recent years a sensible presumption that they should be adjusted in line with the movement in prices from one year to the next' (House of Commons, 1982, col. 742). Similar statements were made in other budgets, but the Chancellor did not adopt any of the indexation schemes described in Chapter 3, even though such mechanisms had become an accepted part of the direct tax system.

There is little evidence that lobby pressure affected major budget decisions made by Chancellor Howe. Indeed the period saw an increasing use of press leaks prior to budgets to build up expectations of large tax changes which might defuse lobby criticism in the event of a smaller change. There were large and frequent increases in tobacco taxes, but there is no evidence that these were influenced by lobby pressure from health groups. There was, however, some recognition of trade and political pressure on behalf of the Scotch Whisky industry. In 1982 the increase in spirits duty was stated to be low because of representations from industry and constituency interests (House of Commons, 1982, col. 743).

To summarise, revenue objectives would seem to be the major determinant of budget policy between 1979 and 1983. The large tax changes that occurred may have been accompanied by health gains, but there is no evidence of a consistent policy in which health considerations played a major role.

Nigel Lawson, 1984 – 1988

The economic policy of the second term of the Conservative administration was broadly similar to that of the first period of office. There were, however, considerable changes in general economic conditions and, especially towards the end of the second term, tax revenues were buoyant.

In Table 5.7 it can be seen that there were fewer increases, especially for alcohol duties, during this period. Spirits duties, in particular, fell in real value. In contrast, tobacco duties were raised substantially in 1984 and 1986. Another special feature of these changes was the fall in wine duties in 1984. The government had stated that excise taxes should be annually increased in line with inflation, but the figures in Tables 5.7 and 5.8 indicate that this objective was not fulfilled.

Table 5.7

Annual changes in excise tax rates and retail prices, 1984–88, (%)

Year of budget	RPI (March to March)	Beer	Wines	Spirits	Cider	Cigarettes
1984	5.2	11.1	−19.9	1.9	47.4	14.4
1985	6.1	7.5	8.3	1.9	10.6	8.1
1986	4.2	0.0	0.0	0.0	0.0	12.8
1987	4.0	0.0	0.0	0.0	0.0	0.0
1988	3.5	4.7	4.5	0.0	9.7	3.7

Notes and sources: See Table 5.3.

Table 5.8

Changes in the prices and tax incidence for typical products as a result of budgets, 1984–88

Year of budget	Beer (pint)	Whisky (bottle)	Wines (bottle)	Cigarettes (20)
a) Change in typical price (%)				
1984	3	1	−8	8
1985	1	1	4	5
1986	0	0	0	7
1987	0	0	0	0
1988	1	0	1	3
b) Duty and VAT as % price				
1984	38.9	74.9	39.0	74.6
1985	38.6	74.1	41.7	74.6
1986	36.3	72.1	44.8	75.4
1987	35.1	71.8	39.6	74.2
1988	34.7	70.2	39.5	74.0

Post budget prices were estimated using appropriate price indices.
See Table 5.4 for details of calculations.

Sources: See Table 5.4.

Revenue objectives would seem to be important in influencing the decisions of this Chancellor. Inflation proofing excise duties was seen in terms of maintaining the real level of revenue. For example, in 1984 he stated 'the changes in excise duties will, all told, bring in some £840 million in 1984–5, some £200 million more than is required to keep pace with inflation' (House of Commons, 1984, col. 302).

Clearly the overall level of revenue from alcohol and tobacco was the main concern of the Chancellor, but in setting tax rates for individual goods he would seem to have attributed changes to particular lobby or health department pressure. In 1984, for example, health representations were referred to when explaining the large increase in tobacco duties (Hansard, 1984, col. 301). Duty levels were restored to the 1965 levels, but no reason was given for this particular benchmark. In 1986 the cigarette tax increases, which were appreciably higher than was needed to keep pace with inflation, were justified by the statement 'in light of the representations that I have received on health grounds' (House of Commons, 1986, col. 180). In contrast, health concerns for alcohol were not acknowledged and the 1986 cigarette tax hike was not accompanied by changes in alcohol duties. No reason was given for these decisions which on health grounds are inconsistent, but the Chancellor noted that the overall effect of excise changes on petrol and tobacco were expected to raise the same amount of revenue as would have resulted from increasing all the excise duties in line with inflation.

Among the trade lobbies, it is only the Scotch whisky industry that may have felt successful in influencing Chancellor Lawson's budget decisions. Duty levels were allowed to fall in real terms and in 1985 there was specific mention of the difficulties facing the industry and of its importance for Britain's export trade (House of Commons, 1985, col. 799).

The other major factor which directly influenced budget decisions during the period from 1984 was the impact of European Community (EC) regulations. In 1984, the Chancellor reduced wine duties by an amount equivalent to 18p a bottle and increased beer duties by an amount equivalent to 2p a pint (Table 5.8). These changes were made to comply with the European Court ruling that beer and wine were like products and should be taxed at similar rates according to strength of alcohol per volume (Godfrey and Powell, 1985). The influence of EC policies on UK budget decisions may become increasingly important as negotiations on tax harmonisation and the internal market progress. Another possible example of this effect occurred in 1986 when no increase was imposed on cigars and pipe tobacco which according to the Chancellor 'are more heavily taxed here than in most comparable countries' (House of Commons, 1986, col. 180).

Finally, the effect of political cycles was also evident when in 1987 neither alcohol nor tobacco duties were changed in the pre-election Budget. The surprise with which both the health and trade lobby responded to this Budget reflects the Chancellor's success in creating the general belief that duty is inflation proofed, despite the fact that the indexation rule has rarely been followed.

CONCLUSION

All three Chancellors during the period 1974 to 1978 would seem to have been principally concerned with revenue yield when considering changes in alcohol and tobacco duties. Duty changes are, therefore, mainly affected by macroeconomic policies. Chancellors have also exploited the flexible nature of the alcohol and tobacco duties. As long as these duties have such a useful role, it would be difficult to introduce a health policy which required regular increases in tax rates.

There is some evidence that lobbies have influence, particularly in the case of the Scotch whisky industry. As suggested above, however, most health and trade lobbies take the view that, despite chancellors' statements concerning the effects of representations, their influence is small relative to other factors. Government's relationships with alcohol and tobacco producer groups extend beyond their tax lobbying activities. These relationships and the ways that they impede the development of prevention policies are examined in Chapter 6. Parliamentary and public opinion would not seem to be a major direct influence on budget strategy, although their perceived views may act as a constraint on the size of budget changes.

Political cycles and inflation were common features which seem to influence chancellors' decisions and such factors act as impediments to a consistent health policy. In periods of high inflation, for example, there are considerable constraints on a chancellor's ability to index alcohol and tobacco duties for fear of fuelling, or being seen to fuel, the inflation process. Similarly, chancellors face considerable pressure to avoid unpopular budget changes before elections.

Despite the common features of the budgets in the period under study, there are significant differences between the policies of Labour and Conservative governments which have implications for potential health policies. In particular, the Labour administration was concerned about distributional effects when changing taxes on alcohol and tobacco. However, the political climate has shifted considerably and any future Labour government's policies may not exhibit similar characteristics.

Whichever party is in power, chancellors have sought to extract revenue from alcohol and tobacco taxes whilst doing the least political damage. For example, the effectiveness of the Scotch whisky industry lobby may be enhanced by the difficult political position in Scotland for the Conservatives and the key position of the industry in the economy of the region. The lobby might not be so effective if a Labour government were in power. The spirits industry also plays an important part in the actual collection of excise duties for the Government, and although this incurs costs to them, their demands on the government to alleviate the situation are moderated.

The impediments to using tax policy to control consumption of alcohol and tobacco goods arise from the complexity of the budget policy process. The competing interests of the health and trade lobbies have not influenced chancellors' decision making in a pluralistic fashion. Any concessions that chancellors have made to either lobby have merely justified preconceived decisions about alternative objectives, usually revenue raising. The wider economic and political context in which fiscal policy is formulated produces the major impediments to controlling consumption through tax. The move towards tax harmonisation within the EC may further limit the ability to use tax as a means of controlling alcohol and tobacco consumption. These impediments can only be overcome within the present system if both public and parliament appreciate the implications of alcohol and tobacco consumption more fully.

References

Action on Alcohol Abuse, (1986), *An Agenda for Action on Alcohol*, Action on Alcohol Abuse, London.

Alcohol Concern, (1987), *The Drinking Revolution*, Alcohol Concern, London.

Brewers Society, (1986), *Brewing Review*, No. 15, January.

Central Policy Review Staff, (1979), *Alcohol Policies*, Socioligska Institutionen, Stockholm.

DHSS, (1977), *Prevention and Health*, Cmnd. 7074, HMSO, London.

DHSS, (1981), *Drinking Sensibly*, HMSO, London.

Godfrey, C. and Powell, M., (1985), 'Alcohol and tobacco taxation: barriers to a public health perspective', *The Quarterly Journal of Social Affairs*, 4, 329–353.

House of Commons, (1974), 'Budget statement', *Parliamentary Debates 1973–74*, Vol. 871, 5th Series, col. 277–329.

House of Commons, (1976), 'Budget statement', *Parliamentary Debates 1975–76*, Vol. 909, 5th Series, col. 232–282.

House of Commons, (1980), 'Budget statement', *Parliamentary Debates 1979–80*, Vol. 981, 5th Series, col. 1437–1490.

House of Commons, (1982), 'Budget statement', *Parliamentary Debates 1981–82*, Vol. 19, 6th Series, col. 726–757.

House of Commons, (1984), 'Budget statement', *Parliamentary Debates 1983–84*, Vol. 56, 6th Series, col. 286–305.

House of Commons, (1986), 'Budget statement', *Parliamentary Debates 1985–86*, Vol. 94, 6th Series, col. 166–184.

Leedham, W., (1987), 'Data Note 10, Alcohol, tobacco and public opinion', *British Journal of Addiction*, 82, 935–940.

Leigh, M., (1976), *Mobilising Consent: Public Opinion and American Foreign Policy*, Greenwood Press, Westport.

Marsh, A., and Matheson, J., (1983), *Smoking Attitudes and Behaviour*, HMSO, London.

Medical Colleges, (1987), 'Consensus statement on a better response to alcohol related problems prepared at a meeting held on 6th November 1987', Royal College of Psychiatrists, London.

Public Expenditure Committee, (1977), *First Report from the Expenditure Committee, Session 1976 –77: Preventive Medicine*, HMSO, London.

Royal College of Physicians, (1971), *Smoking and Health Now*, Pitman Medical, London.

Sunday Times, (1983), 4 January, 4.

The Times, (1982), 19 January, 3.

Weir, R., (1984), 'Obsessed with moderation: the drinks trades and the drink question', *British Journal of Addiction*, 79, 93–107.

Wood, D., (1986), *Beliefs about Alcohol*, Health Education Council, London.

6 Alcohol and tobacco: the politics of prevention

ROB BAGGOTT

The prevention of ill-health has an important political dimension. Yet surprisingly this dimension has frequently been overlooked in the past. The result has often been a general lack of awareness about the political context amongst those seeking to promote health through prevention. In many cases this has proved costly and the failure to recognise and overcome political obstacles has seriously inhibited the emergence of preventive health strategies.

However, in recent years the signs point to a growing awareness of the politics of prevention. This has occurred particularly in areas where those concerned about public health have foundered on the hard rock of commercial interest as in the case of food policy, lead in petrol, and of course, alcohol and tobacco. Such cases illustrate one method of discovering political obstacles which is head-on collision. There are, however, other less painful and more effective ways of surveying the political environment.

In this chapter the prevention of alcohol and tobacco related problems is examined from a political science perspective. This involves an assessment of the significance of prevention issues in terms of the major actors and institutions in the political system, such as national and local politicians, political parties, the machinery and personnel of central government, pressure groups and the media and public opinion. Finally, by way of conclusion, the prospects for policy change will be summarised in the light of the preceding analysis.

117

POLITICIANS

Perhaps the most appropriate place to begin is with politicians. Many national politicians, that is Members of Parliament (MPs) and active members of the House of Lords, have an interest in alcohol and tobacco in two related senses. On the one hand they have established links with alcohol and tobacco interests and, on the other, they have become interested and involved in alcohol and tobacco issues.

Parliamentary activity, such as questions and debates, often reflects pressure by outside organisations. A few examples illustrate this point. The anti-smoking group Action on Smoking and Health (ASH) communicates with MPs through a parliamentary group which boasts a membership of around one hundred MPs. Action on Alcohol Abuse (AAA) uses a similar channel; the Parliamentary Alcohol Policy and Services Group which has approximately fifty members. The drink industries also have liaison committees, in the form of the All Party Group on Scotch Whisky, and the Wine and Spirits Liaison Committee.

The tobacco and alcohol industries also monitor parliament and keep in touch with a pool of sympathetic MPs. This pool might include MPs with constituency interests in alcohol and tobacco production such as the MPs for Bristol and Nottingham (tobacco), Burton on Trent (brewing) and Banff (Scotch Whisky). Other MPs have a more direct economic interest in the industry. Ivan Lawrence, the MP for Burton is also the director of a brewery. Some MPs are retained as consultants by the tobacco and drinks industries. Neil Hamilton MP is currently employed in this capacity by the Brewers Society. The number of MPs with such interests is often difficult to calculate as many fail to declare their outside interests. Nevertheless, a rough estimate can be made and this puts the number of 'tobacco industry' MPs at one hundred and the number of 'alcohol' MPs at around fifty (*The Times,* 1981; Action on Alcohol Abuse, 1987).

The contacts and channels described above are useful for both lobbies as a means of monitoring parliamentary opinion and influencing the views of backbench MPs. This is particularly important since, as we shall see later, alcohol and tobacco issues cut across party lines. This gives MPs much more scope for independent action as they are less constrained by party discipline. Parliament is also an important forum because of its high profile. By sponsoring parliamentary activities, publicity can be gained and this may have a long term impact on the political agenda (Ingle and Tether, 1981).

It should not be forgotten however that the parliamentary timetable is effectively dominated by the government of the day. This limits the ability of the ordinary backbench MP to shape policy. Those wishing to influence alcohol and tobacco policy therefore generally have to seek the support of ministers. Ministers' views, judgements and support have in practice been crucial to the development of alcohol and tobacco prevention policies. In the 1960s, for example, a succession of positive initiatives by both Conservative and Labour Transport Ministers, Ernest Marples, Tom Fraser and Barbara Castle, secured the introduction of tougher measures to tackle drinking and driving (Baggott, 1988a). In the early 1970s Sir Keith (now Lord) Joseph initiated a number of important developments in alcohol policy including the central funding of voluntary alcohol services (Baggott, 1986b).

Individual ministers can have much influence over the course of policy, but usually require the support of their colleagues. Barbara Castle needed Prime Minister Wilson's support to overcome opposition by other ministers to the breathalyser during the 1960s (Castle, 1976, p.114). On several occasions, however, this kind of support has not been forthcoming. For example, Sir George Young and Patrick Jenkin, Health Ministers in the first Thatcher Government, were thwarted in their attempts to take stronger action on both smoking and alcohol abuse largely because of the lack of support given to them by their Cabinet colleagues (Baggott, 1987a; Taylor, 1984).

It is difficult to explain simply how ministers' views are shaped. Pressure from parliament, pressure groups and the media may well influence ministers' views. One might also speculate on the degree to which personal experience of smoking and drinking influences ministers' perceptions. It is worth noting that Kenneth Robinson, an inveterate smoker, supported the banning of cigarette advertising on TV. A related and often overlooked point concerns the extent to which participation within government, and the stress levels involved, can give rise to anti-social habits. The former civil servant Clive Ponting (1986, p.43) has noted that 'after adrenalin alcohol is probably the major lubricant of Whitehall, and some Ministers crack under the influence'.

So far we have been talking about national politicians. Given the supremacy of Parliament within the British political system it is not surprising that we should focus mainly upon the national level. However, we should not forget that local level prevention activities can be important (Tether and Robinson, 1986). Local councillors, for example, are in a position to influence alcohol and tobacco policy. In Scotland councillors sit on local licensing boards which are responsible for granting liquor licences. They therefore have the potential to regulate the availability of alcohol, although in practice this potential may not be fully exploited. There is also considerable scope for local action on alcohol south of the border. Coventry City Council recently announced plans to introduce a bye-law banning drinking in public places.

Smoking policies can also be shaped by local action. Councillors in Glasgow recently approved a range of measures and initiatives with the intention of making the city a smoke-free zone by the year 2000. Similar anti-smoking campaigns have since been launched by other councils, including some English authorities such as Leicester City Council. Clearly, such examples illustrate that we should not underestimate the ability of local politicians to initiate and promote policies aimed at tackling alcohol abuse and smoking.

Party politics

Politicians, whether local or national, tend to act mainly in accordance with party cues. In parliament MPs are subject to party discipline, enforced by the whip system. Dissension by backbench MPs against party leadership, though tolerated in isolated cases, can ultimately lead to expulsion from the party. At the very least persistent dissent can damage the backbench member's chances of a ministerial career.

As has been already noted, alcohol and tobacco issues cut across party lines. Individual MPs are much more independent on cross-party issues. Because of the uncertainties involved in legislating on cross-party issues, governments tend to avoid legislation in those kinds of areas except where there is strong public and parliamentary support for particular policies. This explains the general lack of legislation on alcohol and tobacco matters with the notable exception of drinking and driving legislation and the recent licensing law reforms. It is worth noting that on both issues the Government perceived a great deal of parliamentary support for such measures (Baggott, 1987c; 1988a).

But although it is generally true that alcohol and tobacco issues cut across, rather than reinforce, party lines it would be wrong to say that the political parties have totally ignored these issues. A measure of party interest in alcohol and tobacco has been demonstrated by the content of recent election manifestoes. For example the 1987 SDP/Liberal Alliance election manifesto contained a commitment to ban tobacco advertising. Current official Labour Party policy also supports such a ban, though it should be noted that a pledge along these lines was removed at a late stage from the 1983 Labour Manifesto for electoral reasons. The 1987 Conservative manifesto on the other hand contained a commitment to relax licensing hours. The Party's success at the polls led to the early introduction of a licensing bill which has now become law.

Even so, this level of interest is a far cry from the situation at the turn of the century when alcohol was a major party political and electoral issue. Then, the main parties were closely aligned with the interests involved with the Liberals being the party of temperance and the Tories the guardian of the drinks trades (Baggott, 1986b). The drink industry and the tobacco industries still generally prefer Conservative governments to those of any other political colour. This is partly because of the Conservatives' support for big business in general but, in the case of the brewers, there is a traditional link with the party. This is perhaps reinforced by the financial contributions made to the Conservative Party by the brewers and also by the distillers. In 1981 for example the twelve drinks firms donated £96,000, approximately 5 per cent of the party's income from company donations (Baggott, 1987, p.175). Nevertheless, alcohol and tobacco issues do not cut evenly across party lines. It is generally true that the centre parties and Labour have a lower opinion of the drinks and tobacco industries and are perhaps less open than the Conservatives to influence from this lobby. But it would be wrong to claim that alcohol and tobacco issues provoke major divisions of opinion between the major parties.

The machinery of government

According to Crossman, political parties are the 'battering rams of change' (Crossman, 1972, p.19). But often parties' intentions are blunted, on achieving office, by the machinery of government. Thus, even if the major parties adopted alcohol and tobacco prevention policies, there is no guarantee that, once in government, coherent strategies would begin to emerge. Indeed, there is a great deal of literature on the difficulties faced by party politicians in getting their policies adopted and implemented. In particular the obstruction of policies by civil servants is a regular feature of Ministerial memoirs (Crossman, 1975; Castle, 1980; Barnett, 1982).

Looked at from a different perspective however, civil service support for policies can be effective in getting ministers to adopt new initiatives. It is well known that civil servants try to sell policies to ministers, as part of their role as policy advisers. For example in the 1960s Health Ministers were advised by their senior medical officers to ban cigarette advertising on TV (Baggott, 1987b, p.138). The advice and support of the medical civil servants at the Department of Health and Social Security (DHSS) was also a crucial factor in the higher profile of alcohol policies in the 1970s (Baggott, 1986a, p.475). Moreover, if the attitudes of senior civil servants can be influenced by outside groups, this opens up a useful channel which such groups may use to shape government policy.

Civil service advice to ministers is generally rooted in what is called the departmental view. This means that, as shown in Chapter 4, Treasury Ministers receive advice which places a high premium on financial matters. As Joel Barnett, a former Treasury Minister, has commented: 'When you are looking at the economy as a whole you can't be concerned with only one aspect of it as serious as the health one is. The trouble is you are always looking at the short term in the Treasury at how you can get the maximum amount of revenue' (*The Listener,* 1980).

Different departments look at alcohol and tobacco in different ways. Each views policy issues from a particular departmental perspective and its civil servants advise ministers accordingly. The outcome of this process is that the DHSS has usually been in a minority when alcohol and tobacco related matters such as taxation, changing the licensing laws, and restricting the promotion of these products, have been considered by government as a whole. As a result there has been much interdepartmental conflict between DHSS and the Ministry of Agriculture, Fisheries and Food (MAFF) and the Department of Trade and Industry (DTI) which respectively sponsor the alcohol and tobacco industries and other departments such as the Treasury and Employment, which have interests that may not be served by reducing alcohol and tobacco consumption. Another problem facing the DHSS has been that it does not directly control a number of key policy instruments, including alcohol and tobacco taxation, which is the responsibility of the Treasury and Customs and Excise (Tether and Harrison, 1988). The most the DHSS can do is make representations to these departments, arguing for increased taxes on health grounds. Though this advice is occasionally taken, the revenue departments are very powerful within government, particularly on spending and taxation matters (Heclo and Wildavsky, 1974; Sandford and Robinson, 1983; see also Chapter 4 of this volume).

In view of the different departmental interests involved, it is perhaps not surprising that the DHSS has been frequently defeated in its attempts to prevent alcohol and tobacco problems. As long ago as 1957 the Cabinet decided against allowing the Health Minister to make a public statement on the risks of smoking (*Daily Telegraph,* 1988). The DHSS has also been defeated on many occasions in Cabinet and departmental committees. During the 1960s legislation on smoking was blocked by the Future Legislation Committee (Taylor, 1984, p.84–85). In the early 1970s, Ministers were advised by an interdepartmental committee of officials not to take strong measures against smoking in view of the economic implications of such action (Taylor, 1984, p.71–2).

Concern about the continuing weakness of the DHSS within the machinery of central government, along with worries about the fragmented responsibility and accountability within Whitehall over alcohol and tobacco matters, has fuelled demands that one department or agency should be given the responsibility for all aspects of alcohol and tobacco. Alternatively, as the Central Policy Review Staff (CPRS) suggested in the case of alcohol, a special Advisory Council could be set up to coordinate policy (CPRS, 1982, p.86; Harrison, 1986).

The present Government has rejected calls for greater coordination in respect of both alcohol and tobacco policy, claiming that well-established arrangements already exist to inform government departments of mutual concerns and to coordinate and implement policy (DHSS, 1981, p.66). Recently however, growing concern over alcohol related problems has led the Government to set up a Ministerial Committee to review and coordinate policy (Home Office, 1987). It remains to be seen whether or not this initiative will be effective in resolving the underlying interdepartmental conflicts which exist.

PRESSURE GROUPS: THE INDUSTRIAL LOBBIES

Pressure groups are a key feature of the political environment. Rival groups compete for the attentions of the policy makers in the hope that their preferred policy will be adopted by government. But pressure groups do not have equal ability to influence policy and some are more powerful than others.

Pressure group power depends on a range of factors. Coherent organisation and good leadership are important. Good political contacts with politicians, government departments, political parties and the media are also useful. The social and economic status of groups and the popular support they command are perhaps the most important factors in achieving success. But one should not forget that the intensity of a group's support on a particular issue is crucial. If a powerful group does not feel strongly about a particular policy issue, then it may be no more influential than a weak group that feels strongly about the same issue.

But pressure groups rarely act alone. In practice they form lobbies - coalitions of groups - in an attempt to broaden the level of support for their case. In the area of alcohol and tobacco policies it is therefore possible to speak of the alcohol lobby, the tobacco lobby and the health lobby. It is also possible to evaluate the power of these lobbies in terms of their all-important economic status. Both the alcohol and tobacco lobbies are powerful commercial lobbies with considerable economic leverage. This is clearly illustrated in the table below.

The economic leverage implied by the figures in the table reinforces the political leverage of these industries and facilitates both political contacts and good organisation.

As we saw earlier, both the alcohol and tobacco industries maintain contact with a number of individual MPs. The alcohol industry has an added advantage because of its historical ties with the Conservative Party. The alcohol and tobacco industries are also in continuous and close contact with a number of government departments. They are particularly close to their

Table 6.1

Economic leverage of the alcohol and tobacco industry

	Alcohol	Tobacco
No. of companies in top 50 largest	4	3
Profits before tax (£m)	1300	814
UK employment (000)	512	16.9
Indirect taxation as % of exchequer revenue	4.5	4.1
Exports (% of visible exports)	1.8	0.5
Proportion of consumer spending	7.4	3.3

Sources: Company Reports: The Times Top 1000 Companies: Central statistical Office
UK National Accounts; Department of Employment Employment Gazette,
Department of Trade and Industry Overseas Trade Statistics. Figures for
1986.

sponsoring departments - the drinks industry with MAFF and the tobacco industry with the DTI. These departments will often defend the industry during interdepartmental discussions on alcohol and tobacco related matters. The industries also have a great deal of contact with other departments including the Treasury, Customs and Excise and, in the case of the drinks industry, the Home Office which has the lead responsibility for liquor licensing issues. The industries are also in contact with the DHSS on the health and social aspects of alcohol and tobacco use. Indeed the tobacco industry has built up a close relationship with this department as a result of the regular renegotiation of the voluntary agreements which regulate non-broadcast advertising in all its forms (Baggott, 1987b).

Both the alcohol and tobacco industries, in view of their economic leverage and political contacts can be regarded as 'insider' interests. They are accepted by government as legitimate organisations to be consulted when policy is being decided. This is a considerable advantage and according to some commentators this can, in some situations, confer a veto power over policy (Popham, 1981; Calnan, 1984). Most of the alcohol and tobacco industries' contact with government is through the producers' and importers' trade associations such as the Brewers Society, the Scotch Whisky Association, the Wines and Spirits Association; and in the case of tobacco, the Tobacco Advisory Council (TAC) and the Imported Tobacco Products Advisory Council (ITPAC). Retailers' organisations with an interest in alcohol and/or tobacco, such as the National Union of Licensed Victuallers, the British Hotels Caterers and Restaurants Association, the British Retailers

Association and the Retail Confectioners and Tobacconists' Association also make representations to government, though they are generally less influential than the producers (Baggott, 1987a, pp.138–186; 1987b).

The alcohol and tobacco lobbies are well organised to oppose policies suggested by the health lobby. In the case of alcohol the Brewers Society has adopted an informal lead role as spokesman for the drinks industry on alcohol related problems. This is largely because it stands to lose most from restrictions on alcohol. Unlike the spirits industry it produces mainly for the domestic market. Also within the domestic alcohol market, beer is the largest sector accounting for around half of the expenditure on alcoholic drink. However it should be emphasised that the brewers have diversified into other alcohol sectors such as wines, spirits and cider and other products, and into retail and leisure services, partly in an attempt to reduce their vulnerability to any restrictions in the UK alcohol market. The tobacco lobby is led by the TAC. Again, the aim is to present a united and coherent viewpoint on the health issue thus enhancing the influence of the lobby as a whole.

Both the alcohol and tobacco lobbies have attempted to enlist the support of other industrial groups. These include suppliers of raw materials such as the farmers who supply barley and hops to the drinks industry. Around 20 per cent of the British barley output and around two thirds of domestic hop production are used each year by UK brewers and distillers. This represents a significant economic interest by farmers in the fortunes of the industry, accounting as it does for 6 per cent of the value of crop production. Another industry whose fortunes are linked to alcohol is the advertising industry. Alcoholic drink advertisements account for 4.2 per cent of advertising revenue. Most of this is in the form of television advertising. The Independent Broadcasting Authority (IBA) has estimated that around 7 per cent of its revenue comes from drinks advertisements. The advertising industry also depends to some extent on the tobacco industry though tobacco advertising expenditure is lower - accounting for 1.5 per cent of press and TV spending. However, this figure excludes poster advertising, a major form of tobacco promotion.

Other groups are also enlisted to support the alcohol and tobacco lobbies. These include consumer organisations such as the Campaign for Real Ale (CAMRA), the Freedom Organisation for the Right to Enjoy Smoking Tobacco (FOREST), trade unions such as the General and Municipal Workers Union and the Transport and General Workers (which together have 50,000 members in brewing and distilling), the National Union of Licensed House Managers (around 10,000 members) and the Tobacco Workers Union (around 12,000 members).

Finally we turn to the question of intensity. The drinks industry, which has not diversified into other products to the same extent as the tobacco industry, appears to have a more intense interest in opposing the health lobby. Around 70 per cent of the larger brewers' profits are from alcohol, considerably more than the 42 per cent which the largest tobacco companies derive from tobacco. Even so the tobacco industry still finds tobacco very profitable and this strengthens its desire to fight anti-smoking policies. To conclude then, both industries have a great deal to lose by backing down on the health issues and a lot to gain by standing firm. They have, moreover, the resources - economic, political and organisational—with which to do this.

THE HEALTH LOBBIES

Those who are campaigning for action on alcohol and smoking have no economic leverage. But the anti-smoking and anti-alcohol lobbies do nevertheless contain groups which have considerable social status. The British Medical Association (BMA) and the Royal Colleges of Medicine carry a great deal of weight both in the eyes of the general public and within government. These medical organisations have used a combination of 'insider' and 'outsider' strategies in their attempts to promote government action in respect of alcohol and tobacco consumption. The periodic reports by certain Royal Colleges on smoking and alcohol abuse (Royal College of Physicians, 1962, 1977, 1983, 1987; Royal College of Psychiatrists, 1979, 1986; Royal College of General Practitioners, 1986)—along with high profile public campaigns by the BMA on smoking (BMA, 1986a)—have attracted a lot of public attention and have made the political climate more sympathetic to government intervention. At the same time close contact between the BMA, the Royal Colleges and the Health Departments has provided a useful means for influencing health policy (Baggott, 1987a, p.97–9; 1987b, p.138).

The medical organisations are clearly involved in both alcohol and tobacco issues. To an extent this can be seen as a weakness in that the efforts of these groups are torn between two campaigns. One has to remember that a group's resources are finite; the more campaigns it is involved in, the more thinly spread its resources will be, and all other things being equal, the less effective each individual campaign. As a result the intensity of pressure and involvement along the range of policy issues may be lowered.

The medical organisations are aware of this problem. This partly explains why the Royal College of Physicians (RCP) during the 1970s was not keen to extend its periodic reports on smoking and health to cover alcohol abuse. Instead the Faculty of Community Physicians within the RCP produced its own report (Faculty of Community Medicine, 1980) but this did not achieve anything like the publicity of the Royal College's smoking and

126

health reports. The BMA has also tended to focus on one campaign at a time. In the 1960s and 1970s most of the BMA's efforts went into campaigning for restrictions on drinking and driving. In the 1980s it has become more involved in the anti-smoking campaign and the issue of children and alcohol (BMA, 1986a; 1986b).

Partly because of the difficulties in keeping up constant and intense pressure on a range of alcohol and tobacco related issues, the medical organisations decided to create permanent anti-smoking and anti-alcohol campaigning bodies. ASH was created in 1971 by the Royal College of Physicians and now attracts funding from the DHSS, a sign that, for the present at least, it is seen by that Department as a legitimate campaigning body. A similar function in the alcohol field is performed by Action on Alcohol Abuse. 'Triple A' was founded under the auspices of the Royal Medical Colleges in 1982. However, unlike ASH it does not attract DHSS funding and its resources are therefore even more limited. In the case of alcohol, the campaign has been assisted by the support of bodies such as Alcohol Concern, the government funded national voluntary body for alcohol abuse, and the Health Education Council (HEC) now replaced by a new agency, the Health Education Authority.

A range of other groups is also concerned with alcohol and tobacco. The temperance organisations and associated organisations, such as the Institute for Alcohol Studies (IAS) and the Churches Council on Alcohol and Drugs (CCAD), are active campaigners. The health lobbies can draw on support from a wider range of groups on more specific issues. For example, the Royal Society for the Prevention of Accidents (RoSPA) and the motoring organisations, such as the Royal Automobile Club (RAC) and the Automobile Association (AA), have joined in the campaigns against drinking and driving since the early 1970s (Baggott, 1988a).

The anti-alcohol lobby contains more groups than the anti-smoking lobby. But it is at the same time more fragmented and this is a source of weakness. Also both lobbies suffer from a lack of resources compared with their industrial counterparts.

Even so, in terms of political contacts with MPs and government departments, the health lobby does not fare too badly. As we saw earlier, effective contact has been made through backbench groups and the like. Within government itself however the health lobby is focused almost wholly on the Health Departments. It does not have the wide range of contacts within Whitehall enjoyed by the drink and tobacco industries. Given the relatively low status of the Department of Health within central government, and the fact that it is often outnumbered by other departments on alcohol and tobacco issues, this is clearly a problem for these lobbies.

Health groups have, however, recognised this problem and have attempted to influence other departments directly. For example, the BMA has had contact with the Home Office and the Department of Transport on the subject of drinking and driving in the past (Baggott, 1988a). More recently, in 1986, the Royal Colleges and the BMA had a joint meeting with the Treasury in an attempt to promote an increase in taxation on cigarettes (*British Medical Journal,* 1986). By putting pressure on other departments in this way, the health lobby seeks both to shape the arguments taking place within central government and strengthen the hands of the Health Departments in Whitehall discussions.

PUBLIC OPINION

Any lobby that wishes to influence government policy has to be well organised and well connected politically. But the lobby must also be able to demonstrate a considerable degree of public support or approval for the policies it is promoting. This is particularly the case where an issue cuts across party lines, and/or where policies will affect a large proportion of the population in a significant way. Alcohol and tobacco policy issues fit into both these categories. Indeed one of the most serious problems faced by the health lobby has been the need to persuade government of the political acceptability of alcohol and tobacco prevention policies. One of the main reasons why this is problematic lies in the incidence of these social habits. Around 90 per cent of the British adult population drink alcohol and around a third smoke (OPCS, 1984; 1985). Policies which seek to reduce smoking and alcohol related problems by restricting the price, use, or availability of these products carry the risk of incurring public hostility on some scale.

But latent hostility to controls is not necessarily an automatic product of consumption or indulgence. Both smokers and drinkers may be prepared to see restrictions on themselves and others such as under-age drinkers, smoking in public places and so on. However, survey evidence indicates that support for government intervention in alcohol and tobacco is fairly limited, particularly when compared with the level of support for action on illicit drugs. In 1984 a Gallup survey asked the general public about the seriousness of drug-related social problems. At that time, 78 per cent of the sample believed illicit drug taking was a very serious problem, compared with 42 per cent who believed drunkenness to be serious and 34 per cent who felt the same was true of heavy smoking (*Gallup,* 1984).

Levels of support for specific alcohol and tobacco prevention policies are mixed. Most post-1975 polls show a small majority approving increased taxation on tobacco (Leedham, 1987). On the other hand, there seems to be a considerable majority against using taxation to discourage alcohol consumption and misuse. The question of an advertising ban on tobacco raises similar sentiments, with over 50 per cent consistently supporting a ban on tobacco advertising with only a small minority supporting a total ban on alcohol advertising, although there is more support for a ban on TV advertising of alcohol (MORI, 1980). There is, however, a great deal of support for drink-driving restrictions. Since the late 1970s there has been an overwhelming majority in favour of stronger measures such as random testing and tougher penalties for offenders (Leedham, 1987). It is also worth noting in this context that strong public support for drink-driving restrictions in the 1960s was a major factor behind the emergence of the breathalyser law in this period (Baggott, 1988a).

Finally, one cannot discuss public opinion without also mentioning the media which has a central role in shaping attitudes and mobilising public opinion. The health lobby has to recognise the extent to which the media may be predisposed against it. Journalists are high on the list of alcohol abusers and some may not want to recognise the problem. More importantly, both the broadcast and non-broadcast media depend to a considerable extent on tobacco and alcohol advertising revenue and this may shape their perspective. In addition, the growing diversification of alcohol companies into broadcasting and cable television should be noted. Whitbread now owns 20 per cent of Television South (Baggott, 1987a, p.217). This kind of development may bolster institutional biases against the recognition and prevention of alcohol and tobacco related problems. Finally one has to be aware of the role of advertising and sports sponsorship generally. All of these are essentially insidious ways of ensuring that alcohol and tobacco are socially acceptable products. But more importantly they serve to reinforce the idea that any attempt to control their use and abuse is unacceptable.

CONCLUSION

The level of public support for alcohol and tobacco prevention policies is crucial to the emergence of such policies. Foreign evidence supports this, as a recent study of the comparative politics of smoking in Norway and the UK clearly shows (Baggott, 1986b). This is why the health lobby, if it is to succeed, has to improve and extend its public image. Above all, it must avoid the adverse image which is produced by the charge that it is dictating lifestyles and curtailing individual freedom. Its public campaigns should, therefore, stress on the one hand the importance of choice, and on the other, freedom from the problems caused by the misuse of alcohol and the use of tobacco.

But such a high public profile should not inhibit an 'insider' strategy, that is, an approach based on close contacts with policy makers. Indeed public support is complementary to such an approach since it should enable health groups to strengthen their contacts with government and parliament, and give the lobbies greater leverage. Moreover, by persuading government to accord a higher priority to these problems, this in turn may feed back on public opinion and could, as a result, increase the level of support for further action on alcohol and tobacco.

The general theme of this review of the actors and institutions with roles in the politics of prevention is clearly one of confrontation. The politics of alcohol and tobacco is best understood from such a perspective given the conflict of interest between the vested economic interests and the health lobby. But does prevention have to be confrontational? It may have to be in the case of tobacco. This is because the ultimate aims of the competing lobbies are mutually incompatible and there is little scope for compromise since the health lobby is trying to prevent use, not abuse. However, the situation is different where alcohol is concerned for there the problem is abuse, not use. The drinks industry has a commercial interest in reducing the level of alcohol misuse which reflects adversely on its product. So, on issues like alcohol education there is considerable scope for consensus and compromise and there may be other possible compromises which remain unexplored.

For the moment though, alcohol appears to be following tobacco down the road of confrontation, particularly where control policies are concerned. Whether this will continue or not remains to be seen. It depends a great deal on the strategies of the lobbies involved and on the relationship between them and government. In principle, therefore, the politics of prevention is not necessarily a zero sum game, though in practice it may remain so.

References

Action on Alcohol Abuse, (1987), *Personal Correspondence.*

Baggott, R., (1986a), 'Alcohol, politics and social policy', *Journal of Social Policy*, 15, 4, 467–88.

Baggott, R., (1986b), *The Politics of Alcohol: Two Periods Compared*, Institute for Alcohol Studies Occasional Paper No. 8, London.

Baggott, R., (1987a), *The Politics of Public Health: Alcohol, Politics and Social Policy*, (University of Hull PhD Thesis, unpublished).

Baggott, R., (1987b), 'Government-industry relations in Britain: the regulation of the tobacco industry', *Policy and Politics*, 15, 3, 137–46.

Baggott, R., (1987c), 'Licensing law reform and the return of the drink question', *Parliamentary Affairs*, 40, 4, 50–16.

Baggott, R., (1988a), 'Drinking and driving: the politics of social regulation', *Teaching Politics*, 17, 1.

Baggott, R., (1988b), *Health v Wealth: The Politics of Smoking in Norway and the UK*, Papers in Politics No. 57, University of Strathclyde, Glasgow.

Barnett, J., (1982), *Inside the Treasury*, Andre Deutsch, London.

British Medical Association, (1986a), *Smoking Out the Barons*, Wiley, Chichester.

British Medical Association, (1986b), *Young People and Alcohol*, BMA, London.

British Medical Journal, (1986), 8 March, Vol. 292, 710

Calnan, M., (1984), 'The politics of health: the case of smoking control', *Journal of Social Policy*, 13, 3, 278–96.

Castle, B., (1976), *The Castle Diaries 1964–70*, Weidenfeld and Nicholson, London.

Castle, B., (1980), *The Castle Diaries 1974–76*, Weidenfeld and Nicholson, London.

Central Policy Review Staff, (1982), *Alcohol Policies in the UK*, Sociologiska Institionen, Stockholm.

Crossman, R.H.S., (1972), *Inside View*, Cape, London.

Crossman, R.H.S., (1975), *The Diaries of a Cabinet Minister*, Hamish Hamilton and Cape, London.

Daily Telegraph, 2nd January 1988, 1.

Department of Health and Social Security, (1981), *Drinking Sensibly*, HMSO, London.

Faculty of Community Medicine, (1980), *A Recommendation for the Prevention of Alcohol Related Disorders*, Royal College of Physicians, London.

Gallup Political Index, (1984), September No. 289.

Harrison, L., (1986), 'Is a coordinated prevention policy really feasible?' *Alcohol and Alcoholism*, 21, 5–6.

Harrison, L. and Tether, P., (1988), *Alcohol Policies: Responsibilities, Relationships in British Government*, Addiction Research Centre, Hull.

Heclo, H. and Wildavsky, A., (1974), *The Private Government of Public Money*, Macmillan, London.

Home Office, (1987), *Press Release*, 18 September.

Ingle, S. and Tether, P., (1981), *Parliament and Health Policy*, Gower, London.

Leedham, W., (1987), 'Data Note 10, Alcohol, tobacco and public opinion', *British Journal of Addiction*, 82, 935–40.

The Listener, (1980), 18– 5 December, 815–17.

Millstone, E., (1986), *Food Additives*, Penguin, Harmondsworth, .

MORI opinion poll, (1980), *Sunday Times*, 18 December, p.1.

Office of Population Censuses and Surveys, (1984), *General Household Survey*, HMSO, London.

Office of Population Censuses and Surveys, (1985), *OPCS Monitor GHS 85/2*, HMSO, London.

Ponting, C., (1986), *Whitehall: Tragedy and Farce*, Hamish Hamilton, London.

Popham, G.T., (1981), 'Government and smoking: policy making and pressure groups', *Policy and Politics*, 9, 3, 331–47.

Royal College of Physicians, (1962), *Smoking and Health*, Pitman, London.

Royal College of Physicians, (1971), *Smoking and Health Now*, Pitman, London.

Royal College of Physicians, (1977), *Smoking or Health?*, Pitman, London.

Royal College of Physicians, (1983), *Health or Smoking?*, Pitman, London.

Royal College of Physicians, (1987), *The Medical Consequences of Alcohol Abuse: A Great and Growing Evil*, Tavistock, London.

Royal College of Psychiatrists, (1979), *Alcohol and Alcoholism*, Tavistock, London.

Royal College of Psychiatrists, (1986), *Alcohol—Our Favourite Drug*, Tavistock, London.

Royal College of General Practitioners, (1986), *Alcohol: a Balanced View*, Reports from General Practice No. 24.
Sandford, C. and Robinson, A., (1983), *Tax Policy Making in the UK*, Heinemann, London.
Taylor, P., (1984), *Smoke Ring*, Bodley Head, London.
Tether, P. and Robinson, D., (1986), *Preventing Alcohol Problems: a guide to local action*, Tavistock, London.
The Times, (1981), 17th November, 2.
Wilson, D., (1983), *The Lead Scandal*, Heinemann, London.

7 Industry and employment policy: department and group relations

PHILIP TETHER AND LARRY HARRISON

Although in overall economic terms the tobacco industry is relatively small, both it and the alcohol industry are very important in terms of revenue and health lobbyists identify economic considerations as the major impediment to the development of effective, coordinated prevention strategies (Alcohol Concern, 1987). One 'economic consideration' is said to be government unwillingness to sacrifice present revenue from the sale of alcohol and tobacco for future health benefits. This claim has been examined in previous chapters which have found that the formation of tax policy in respect of alcohol and tobacco is both more complex than health lobbyists often suppose and less open to the influence of producer groups than they believe. By analysing the tax policy process, specific impediments to prevention were identified, thus clarifying the steps which could be taken to develop a more coordinated prevention strategy. The purpose of this chapter is to provide a similar overview of government/producer relations in the field of industrial and employment policies in respect of alcohol and tobacco.

The overt commitment of government to the well-being of the two industries and their associated interests is not in doubt. A cluster of three major departments—the Department of Trade and Industry (DTI), the Ministry of Agriculture, Fisheries and Food (MAFF) and the Department of Employment (DoEmp) have very specific responsibilities in relation to their economic health and success. The focus is, therefore, on the structure and processes linking government (or at least parts of government) with producer interests, rather than on the substance of those policies.

Two of the departments, the DTI and MAFF, lie at the centre of organisational networks which incorporate the alcohol and tobacco manufacturers and, depending on the issue, other government departments and a variety of non-governmental groups and organisations. The third department, the DoEmp, has a general interest in the economic health and competitiveness of these industries which reinforces the more specific concerns of DTI and MAFF.

The concept of organisational networks is important to an understanding of the relationship between groups and departments not only in respect of alcohol and tobacco policy but also other issues. In a complex world, policy is seldom the complete property and prerogative of a single organisation whether governmental or non-governmental. Increasingly, policy development and implementation are shared between a number of organisations (Hjern and Porter, 1981). Organisations having significant amounts of interaction with each other form policy networks where organisations and issues come together. Sometimes this interaction is based on mutual benefit and a reciprocal exchange of resources, sometimes on conflict or, more usually, on a shifting mixture of the two. Often, organisational linkages are mediated by professionals located in organisational sub-units and these professionals may have more in common with their 'opposite numbers' in other organisations, than with their own colleagues (Friend et al., 1974). Organisations move into, and out of, particular networks according to the policy issue at hand. For this reason, we prefer to use the term policy network rather than the label 'policy community' (Richardson and Jordan, 1979) which tends to imply stability of membership and the existence of consensus. Because peripheral membership may change from issue to issue, clear boundaries cannot be drawn around organisational networks. Moreover, every organisational network has sub-networks where the focus is on specific issues. On any given issue, networks may intersect. Nevertheless, there are typical constellations of organisations and groups concerned with particular sets of related issues and which have more contact with each other than with those in other constellations (Harrison and Tether, 1987).

It is a convention of the conflict-avoiding, consensus-seeking British political system with its tradition of corporate representation (Beer, 1965) that in framing policies 'the appropriate department must consult the appropriate outside *interest*' (Jennings, 1959, p.102). This administrative culture has facilitated and promoted the increasingly close relationship between government and groups which intervention in the economic and social life of the nation has necessitated. Government needs certain groups for information, advice and cooperation in the development and implementation of policy and, in return, these favoured groups receive a measure of influence over policy which affects them. This influence can extend to agenda setting (Richardson and Jordan, 1979) as well as non-decision making and symbolic policy-making (Ham, 1982). In the most favoured cases, groups may be accorded statutory rights to representation on various public or quasi-governmental bodies or, as in the case of farmers, legislation may confer on government an obligation to consult groups where their interests are involved. The result has been a vast extension of pressure group politics, embedded in organisational networks, around functionally differentiated departments. The policy-making process involves departments in reaching agreement with affected groups and then, if necessary, selling the resulting 'package' within government (Norton, 1987). Organisational networks which are 'plugged into' different departments seldom intersect leaving it to internal, governmental processes to reconcile their differences which means that 'government departments whilst often being the target of external pressure groups are also playing pressure group roles themselves' (Richardson and Jordan, 1979, p.25). Thus, representatives of groups and organisations in the health network around the DHSS have virtually no independent contact with the industry network focused on the MAFF, the DTI and the DoEmp and contact between the Health Departments and departments in the producer network can be fraught with difficulties. When Edwina Currie, Junior Health Minister at the Department of Health and Social Security, proposed that the Health and Safety at Work Act 1974, should be used as a vehicle for workplace smoking and alcohol policies she incurred the opposition of the 'dry', libertarian Employment Under Secretary, Patrick Nicholls. One Conservative backbencher saw the proposal as both ideologically distasteful and as infringing departmental autonomy: 'It is bad enough John Moore allowing Nanny Currie to preach to everybody in the DHSS but she has no right to extend this to the Department of Employment' (*The Guardian,* 1988).

The Currie proposal has obvious merits and would open the producer network up to health-oriented considerations, but its reception is not surprising. Saunders (1981) has drawn attention to the preoccupation of national policy makers with production as opposed to consumption issues which, by and large, are devolved to the local government level. Moreover, consumer interests, as opposed to producer interests, are fragmented 'since most men earn their incomes in one area but spend them in many' (Downs, 1957, p.254). Thus, 'numbers are far less important than group organisations' (Richardson and Jordan, 1979, p.173) and, 'possessing such organisations it is producer groups which tend to have the closest contacts and the greatest degree of influence' (Ham, 1982, p.78) with government.

Governments win and lose elections on the management of the economy and the health and welfare of consumers has not been an electoral issue since religion and politics entwined in the Nineteenth Century around the 'drink question'.

Departmental organisation by function can be of two types, both of which were identified at the turn of the century by the Machinery of Government Committee (Haldane Report, 1918). The first is distribution according to the persons or classes to be dealt with and the second, distribution according to the services to be performed. Since the former would lead to a fragmentation of services and the duplication of provision, departmental development has proceeded not along clientele-based lines but according to services performed. Haldane identified ten distinct 'separate' administrations which he believed would cover the range of government services and these included Finance, National Defence, External Affairs, Research and Information, Production, Employment, Supplies, Education, Health and Justice. The DTI, the MAFF and the DoEmp departmental group clearly correspond to Haldane's Production and Employment functions.

The organisation of the British Executive into functionally differentiated departments according to services performed has a number of consequences. First, it is well recognised that each department has its own perspectives on policy and a distinct organisational culture (Greenwood and Wilson, 1984) which gives rise to a variety of centre-local relationships and colours departments' links with peripheral agencies (Griffith, 1966). The result is a high degree of 'departmentalism' in which ministers' success depends 'more on how well they provide for the department in the annual budgetary battles than on policy innovation and experimentation' (Ashford, 1981, p.33). Departmentalism played an important part in blunting attempts to introduce a comprehensive system of public expenditure planning in the 1960s and 1970s. Barbara Castle made the same point when, after joining the Cabinet, she observed: 'I suddenly found I wasn't in a political caucus at all. I was faced by departmental enemies' (*The Sunday Times,* 1973). Departmentalism affects the DTI, MAFF and the DoEmp as much as other departments. Thus, the Industry and Employment departments 'have a considerable tendency towards protectionism' whilst the Department of Trade 'has traditionally been a free trade department' (Williams, 1980, p.89). In 1983, the Departments of Trade and Industry were merged to form the DTI bringing different perspectives and priorities under one organisational roof. Nevertheless, although MAFF, the DTI and the DoEmp are divided by different perspectives and priorities there is much, as this chapter will seek to show, which unites them.

Secondly, organisation by services performed calls for a high degree of intra- and inter-departmental coordination. Coordination can be defined as 'the controlling of activities and decisions of individuals or agencies so that they are harmonised in the pursuit of some stated common goal or objectives' (Stanyer and Smith, 1976, p.157). Within departments, a variety of administrative units such as sections, branches and divisions, have the 'lead responsibility' for specific issues and these act as the focal points of policy development, responding to pressures and demands both from within government and within the networks to which they are connected. All policies have implications for other policies and will usually depend for their implementation on a variety of administrative units located both within and across departments. Intra-departmental coordination is fostered not only by informal links between civil servants within a department but also by the hierarchic structure itself and the functional principle of work allocation which locates related functions within the same departmental divisions (Greenwood and Wilson, 1984, p.39). Between departments, policy coordination is fostered by the network of personal contacts between civil servants at every organisational level (Heclo and Wildavsky, 1981), and by a variety of institutional devices. These include ad hoc, issue-specific, inter-departmental advisory committees (IDACs), the Public Expenditure Survey Committee (PESC) which agrees the costing basis of each department's planned expenditures before they are submitted to political judgement and, finally, the Cabinet, with its sub-structure of Cabinet committees. The prime function of the Cabinet 'is to resolve those issues which cannot be resolved elsewhere' (Burch, 1987, p.27) but in practice such issues are relatively few when measured against the volume of government business.

The main feature of the coordination process is that, at both the intra- and inter-departmental level, it proceeds incrementally (Lindblom, 1965) issue by issue. Moreover, 'stated common goals or objectives', are the property of individual departments or groups of departments if they are linked to one organisational network and share a common concern for a policy issue. This is the case with the DTI, the MAFF, and the DoEmp. The fragmentation of lead responsibilities in respect of alcohol policy was underlined by the Report *Alcohol Policies* (CPRS, 1979) which identified sixteen government departments with a variety of interests in the production, distribution and retailing of potable (i.e. drinkable) alcohol and the many problems associated with its consumption. However, these departments coordinate policy if they share a common concern for a type of issue. Thus, in addition to the production network there are a number of other 'alcohol networks' covering such areas as law and order, health and safety, advertising and the media (where the DTI also appears) education and alcohol agencies of various kinds (Harrison and Tether, 1987) each of which has as its focus either a department or a cluster of departments. Contact across network boundaries between departments representing different kinds of interest is rare because it is unnecessary. Where it occurs, the outcome will be even more political and dependent upon the status and power of the departments involved than is the case within networks.

Thus, a major impediment to the development of comprehensive coordinated prevention strategies for both alcohol and tobacco is the functionally differentiated structure of British government and the lack of inter-network coordinating mechanisms and processes. The recently established Ministerial Group on Alcohol Misuse (Home Office, 1987), which contains Ministers from eleven departments, is the first attempt to facilitate inter-departmental and inter-network coordination of alcohol policy. The DTI, the MAFF and the DoEmp are responsible for the economic interests and well-being of the alcohol and tobacco industries and lie at the focus of the producer networks. The next section outlines the nature of government-producer relations and the organisational structures and processes which foster those relations. The purpose is simple. Calls for coordinated strategies are unlikely to carry much weight until those making them are very clear not only about what should be done, but also what is being done. As previous chapters have shown, it is only by analysing current policies and identifying 'impediments to prevention' that we can bring realistic options into focus.

THE DEPARTMENTS

Ministry of Agriculture, Fisheries and Food (MAFF) The MAFF is formally recognised throughout government as the sponsor for the alcohol industry. Sponsorship is the formalisation and institutionalisation of group-department relationships in which the department assumes specific responsibility for articulating a group's views and interests, for acting as the industry's 'friend at court' and for providing a two-way channel of communication with the black box of government decision-making. Sponsorship does not automatically turn a department into an uncritical advocate of a group's interests when policy is being made, but it does confer on a department a general duty to watch over, guard and defend the welfare of its clients. The doctrine applies most commonly to groups producing goods and services, but the services need not be commercial. The Home Office is the sponsor for the police service in the UK.

MAFF identifies the interests of the alcohol producers and represents them within government. If there are conflicts between parts of the industry, the department attempts to assess the merits of rival points of view and their implications for policy development. MAFF's sponsorship obligations

138

involve the Department in monitoring, regulation and technical assistance. The monitoring function involves identifying policy developments elsewhere in government which might have implications for alcohol producers and importers. For example, if the DHSS were arguing for the adoption of policies aimed at reducing per capita consumption of alcohol, MAFF would be active on behalf of producer interests. A recent example of MAFF's regulatory function was the decision to extend a European Community (EC) Directive (that all bottles and cans of alcoholic drinks should display alcohol content as a percentage of volume) to beer pumps and other drink dispensers in hotels, restaurants and public houses (MAFF, 1987). MAFF offers technical assistance to alcohol producers and government laboratory analysts may be brought in to help resolve scientific problems.

The existence of specific issues affecting different parts of the producer network is reflected in MAFF's internal organisation. The focus of MAFF's responsibility for the potable alcohol industry is its Alcoholic Drinks Division (ADD) which contains two branches. Branch A deals with all aspects of wine. This includes the UK wine trade, the producers of British wine and British sherry (both made in the UK from imported grape juice) and the small but growing native English wine industry. However, the major part of its work is taken up with EC matters. Civil servants from Branch A attend the Community's Special Wine Working Group and its Wine Management Committee, both of which meet weekly. Branch B deals with all other alcoholic drinks including Scotch whisky, gin, vodka, beer and cider. The ADD has close relations with the Ministry's Standards Division and its Food Science Division, which together take the lead on regulating the constituents of alcoholic beverages. Other divisions may occasionally be involved in the development of alcohol policy. One such is the Cereals Division, because large quantities of grain are used in the production of beer, whisky and the neutral alcohol utilised in the manufacture of other drinks. Another is the Horticultural Division, which represents the interests of British hop growers who are suffering from the growing popularity of lager, some of which is manufactured with imported hops.

MAFF has strong links with the DTI over alcohol export policy and both it and the trade departments of the DTI seek to expand exports, increase foreign earnings and reduce tariff barriers where these prevent the development of overseas trade in alcoholic beverages. Contact with the DTI over alcohol trade issues is usually on an ad hoc basis but there are more formal consultations over specific issues, particularly Scotch whisky which is examined in detail in Chapter 9. During the last decade this industry's labour force has fallen from 23,000 to 16,000 and sixteen distilleries have gone out of business. Changing domestic drinking habits have played a part in this decline but the main problem for an industry which depends on exports for 84 per cent of sales revenue has been very high import duties, especially in Japan, where a bottle of Scotch whisky costs about £80. Heavy pressure has been brought to bear on the Japanese to 'end discrimination and allow Scotch to compete fairly with their own brand, Suntory' (*The Daily Telegraph*, 1987). MAFF also has close and continuing contact with Branch 6 of the Revenue Duties Division B (RDB) within HM Customs and Excise. Division B is responsible for duties on alcoholic drinks and Branch 6 is particularly concerned with the rates and structure of alcohol duty, Budget calculations and international questions including EC harmonisation of excise duties. Like MAFF, HM Customs and Excise have close links with the trade.

As the sponsor of the UK alcohol industry, MAFF's main links are with alcohol producers and importers. It has no systematic contact with the distribution and retailing interests which cluster around the alcohol industry, both of which are the DTI's responsibility. However, MAFF is occasionally involved in some retailing issues since the brewers are also retailers through the tied house system. The Federation of Wholesale Distributors, whose principal link is with the DTI, has made representations to MAFF on this subject and on other topics such as a draft EC Directive on Containers of Liquids for Human Consumption.

ADD's links are mainly with trade associations rather than individual companies since it is usually concerned to acquire an industry wide view and it would be too time consuming for the Ministry to canvass individual companies for their opinions. These trade associations include the Scotch Whisky Association, the Wine and Spirits Association, the National Association of Cider Makers, the Gin Rectifiers and Distillers Association, the Vodka Trade Association and the English Vineyards Association. The range of trade associations are a function of the industry's breadth in product terms and each association represents a distinct sub-set of trade interests whose concerns may or may not have implications for each other. The Wine and Spirits Association is the broadest in product terms and it has the largest import interests. The Scotch Whisky Association is, by contrast, predominantly export orientated. There is no umbrella or peak organisation representing the entire alcoholic drinks industry.

The Ministry maintains links with the representative industry groups by letter and telephone and there are regular formal and informal meetings between officials and the trade associations. However, neither the Ministry nor the trade associations are restricted in the range and level of their contacts. Thus, the Ministry attaches considerable importance to maintaining good relations with individual companies and both these companies and their trade associations may on occasion make direct representations to other departments. In such cases, the company or the industry will only enlist the support of MAFF if it was felt that other departments were not giving proper consideration to their views or there was a serious threat to their interests.

Like other British industries, the larger trade associations have representatives in Brussels who monitor EC developments which could have implications for their member companies. Taken in conjunction with the presence of Ministry officials in Brussels and MAFF's monitoring of intra-governmental policies, the trade associations have a sensitive surveillance system capable of detecting possible problems at an early stage.

There is only occasional contact between MAFF and organisations campaigning against alcohol misuse, such as Action on Alcohol Abuse ('Triple A') and the British Medical Association (BMA), whose primary links are with the Department of Health. The BMA has recommended that all drink containers carry a health warning similar to that required on cigarette packets, but it has made no representations to MAFF, the department responsible for food and drink labelling policy. A Working Group of the Standing Conference on Crime Prevention has made a similar suggestion (Home Office, 1987) but the interim list of proposals from the Ministerial Group on Alcohol Misuse does not include any recommendation on this topic (Privy Council, 1988). However, the BMA's views were canvassed by MAFF's Standards Division over its proposed regulations on alcoholic strength labelling. Approximately 150 organisations had an opportunity to comment on the proposals, including the Health Education Authority, the King's Fund Institute, the Medical Council on Alcoholism, the Hops Marketing Board, the Campaign for Real Ale Ltd., and the British Oat and Barley Millers Association.

Department of Trade and Industry (DTI) The DTI is responsible for industrial policy and assistance and it thus has a direct interest in the economic performance of most manufacturing and service industries in the UK apart from a small number such as the manufacturing of alcohol where other departments take the lead responsibility. One of the Department's many areas of responsibility includes the tobacco industry. The organisational focus of its tobacco interests is Branch 2C in the Consumer Market Division. Branch 2C is also responsible for the clothing, footwear and leather industries as well as a number of other commodity groups, and the organisational base of the DTI's tobacco interests is thus very small. Until January 1987, the DTI was the governmental sponsor for the tobacco manufacturers. Before then, the industry side of the Department was divided into ten sponsoring groups which promoted the interests of the industries they covered. These have now been converted into three broad market

141

groups for consumer goods and services (including tobacco), intermediate goods and capital goods. The reorganisation was promoted by Lord Young, the Trade and Industry Secretary, as part of a drive to turn the organisation into the 'DTI-The Department for Enterprise', as it was officially renamed on the 14th January 1987. Sponsorship was felt to be inimical to the development of an entrepreneurial culture. As Lord Young put it: 'For a long time now, the role of the sponsoring department was to act as their spokesman in government. It doesn't work well, so we're ending sponsorship' (*The Sunday Times*, 1988). More specifically the 'enterprise initiative' involves the DTI in the joint funding of consultancies for firms contemplating expansion and the development of new products and services. A few months after the scheme was launched, the Department had received 50,000 applications and was approving grants at the rate of 1,000 a week (*The Sunday Telegraph*, 1988).

The Department's reorganisation and the ending of sponsorship are both designed to counter the allegedly undemanding and essentially reactive stance of the DTI in respect of British industry, the aim being to sharpen the ability of the Department to actively promote enterprise and economic activity. If it works as intended, the end of sponsorship means that industries will find they no longer have an automatically sympathetic 'departmental ear' in government.

Further confirmation of the priority being given to industrial and employment interests comes from the Enterprise and Deregulation Unit (EDU). The EDU is a central task force with staff drawn from a number of government departments and business organisations, charged with pursuing deregulation throughout Whitehall. The unit was created following proposals in two White Papers, *Lifting the Burden* (Cabinet Office, 1985) and *Building Businesses ... not Barriers* (DoEmp, 1986). The EDU was first established in the DTI but followed Lord Young to the Department of Employment. However, with Lord Young's return to the DTI after the General Election of 1987, the EDU has returned to its original location. Most government departments have officers responsible for promoting deregulation and many have their own deregulation units. Each department has to inform the EDU of regulatory proposals, so that any new demands on businesses may be identified. If the Government were proposing a major initiative on alcohol problems which included, for the sake of argument, the extension of licensing controls to wholesale outlets, the relevant department, in this case the Home Office, would notify the EDU. It would also have to estimate the costs and benefits of the proposed regulation, using a seventeen point checklist which, interestingly, does not refer to the health consequences of policy initiatives. The checklist includes questions on whether alternatives to regulation, such as voluntary agreements, have been considered or whether there is any provision for exempting small businesses. Departments are also required to state whether they have engaged in consultation with businesses likely to be affected. If the preliminary assessment does not provide a clear indication of the likely costs to businesses, the EDU may request a cost-benefit analysis, possibly involving surveys of industry. The procedures are intended to ensure that no new regulations are introduced which impose costs on business without clear justification.

The Director of the EDU has the equivalent rank of an Under Secretary. The Unit has two Deputies who are Assistant Secretaries and below them are five Principals. In all, the EDU consists of around twenty staff mostly on short-term secondment. It also has an Advisory Panel on Deregulation, a group of about nine businessmen who act as a 'sounding board', and who advise the Secretary of State on the potential impact of proposed regulation. The EDU has a relatively informal structure, with each Principal being responsible for liaising with a group of departments. The EDU works closely with Branches 4 and 5 in the DTI's General Policy Division. These branches are responsible for the overall development and application of UK competition policy and for liaison with the main competition authorities— the Office of Fair Trading and the Monopolies and Mergers Commission—on its implementation.

Like MAFF, the DTI takes a close interest in the implications of other department's domestic, economic, fiscal and financial politics for the prosperity and health of British industry and constantly monitors policy proposals and developments in other parts of government. Again, like MAFF, taxation policy is a major concern for the DTI. Branch 1 in the DTI's General Policy Division is responsible for formulating the Department's overall position in the annual pre-Budget discussions conducted by HM Customs and Excise when departments with an interest in excise duties (which includes the Department of Health, the MAFF and the DTI) are invited to submit their views. The link in respect of tobacco duties is with Branch 1 of HM Customs and Excise Revenue Duties Division A (RDA), but apart from the annual representations contact is limited. The DTI is not regarded as a particularly effective or energetic advocate of the tobacco industry and the size of the tobacco branch is perhaps indicative of the Department's low level of commitment to a beleaguered and controversial industry. Because of its comprehensive understanding of the impact of fiscal measures on the industry, HM Customs and Excise are sometimes better able than the DTI to articulate and, in effect, represent tobacco interests.

Although the DTI does not have direct responsibility for the potable alcohol industry, many of its interests touch on alcohol-related issues of one kind or another. Thus, it has oversight of firms manufacturing drink processing machinery and of other suppliers to breweries and of the alcohol wholesale and distribution trades. As the promoter of British exports, it provides services and advice to alcohol producers. The Department has four Overseas Trade Divisions and ten Regional Offices throughout the country, working under the guidance of the British Overseas Trade Board (BOTB) which consists mostly of businessmen with experience in aspects of exporting. The DTI's ten Regional Offices are the BOTB's 'front-line' in its relations with exporters and potential exporters. They help exporters by liaising with the appropriate Overseas Trade Division and the commercial departments of the Foreign and Commonwealth Office around the world, by providing information from their own data bases and by supplying information about the financial support which the BOTB offers to encourage market research, trade missions, stands at trade fairs and other activities. An alcohol producer approaching a regional office or an Overseas Trade Division direct would have access to all the information and advice and other services the BOTB can offer, although the company would be advised to contact MAFF for advice on the industry's strategy for exports.

Responsibility for individual countries or groups of countries is divided within the Overseas Trade Divisions between branches, known as Market Branches, which are further sub-divided into sections. A Product Coordination Unit working with Overseas Trade Division 3 (OT3) deals with export matters which are not geographically orientated or which affect products which are the responsibility of other departments. This includes the alcohol industry. The DTI is also responsible for coordinating the UK's input into the external trade policy of the EC. Since accession to the Community, the UK has no independent right to negotiate or enter into international trade agreements. Its contribution to Community trade policy is the responsibility of the DTI's European Policy Division and its International Policy Divisions whose members represent the Department at meetings of Community institutions.

The DTI is also responsible for consumer safety issues, sizes, weights and measures, and sickness and absenteeism, all of which may have an alcohol dimension from time to time. Thus, a section in Branch 4 in the Consumer Affairs Division constitutes a Consumer Safety Unit which, among other things, monitors the Home Accident Surveillance System (HASS) through which data is collected from Accident and Emergency (A and E) departments in England and Wales; a section in Branch 1 in the same division is responsible for prescribing the quantities in which beer and certain spirits may be sold over the bar and the quantities in which still wine may be packed. Branch 2 in the General Policy Division monitors a number of domestic policy areas. These include other departments' policies in relation to sickness and absenteeism which may affect the health and competitiveness

144

of British industry. This Branch would have an important role to play in any future policy initiatives designed to promote the development and spread of alcohol and work policies.

However, one of the Department's most important responsibilities in relation to both alcohol and tobacco involves the advertising industry. The DTI has oversight of this important area of economic activity which had an expenditure of £5117m in 1986 (Waterson, 1987). Branch 2 of the Consumer Affairs Division deals with advertising issues and the DTI strongly favours the current self-regulatory approach to the presentation and content of UK alcohol and tobacco advertising in the broadcast and non-broadcast media, embodied in codes of practice administered by the Independent Broadcasting Authority (IBA) and the Advertising Standards Authority (ASA). The DTI's view of the self-regulatory system—which is regarded as inadequate by many in the public health lobby—is that it is a delicate mechanism which works, and that its replacement by statutory controls would probably be less efficient and less effective.

Unlike the alcohol area, the nature of the product and the industrial structure are such as to provide the Department with one focal point for communication and consultation. The Tobacco Advisory Council (TAC) represents all the UK tobacco manufacturing interests. Another trade organisation, the Imported Tobacco Products Advisory Council (ITPAC), participates in the Department of Health and tobacco industry joint discussions surrounding the regularly re-negotiated voluntary agreements on the advertising and promotion of tobacco products. However, it is very small and there is little contact between it and either the DTI or TAC. Again, as with alcohol, there is regular and continuing contact by letter, telephone and meetings, between Branch 2C and the TAC over issues as they arise. Chief among these are questions involving tobacco taxes and the outcome of these discussions helps to shape the DTI's position in the annual representations it makes to HM Customs and Excise. However, since the TAC is in regular contact with Revenue Duties Division A in Customs and Excise, the DTI usually has little that is new to present at the annual meetings.

The DTI has strong bilateral links with the 'Big 3' tobacco manufacturers (The Imperial Group, Gallaghers and Rothmans) which between them account for about 90 per cent of the UK tobacco market (Booth et al., 1986). Individual companies and the TAC make links with other departments as necessary and one of the strongest is the connection between the TAC and the DHSS over the voluntary agreements on tobacco advertising. The two departments directly involved in forging these agreements are the Department of Health and the Department of Employment (DoEmp) and, although the DTI's views are sought, it does not have a direct role in these negotiations. However, when the DTI discovered that the Department of

145

Health had never held direct talks with advertising interests, they organised a meeting so that advertisers could present their views on the promotion of tobacco products.

Department of Employment (DoEmp)   The third department with a strong interest in the economic performance of the alcohol and tobacco industries is the DoEmp which was formed out of the post-war Ministry of Labour in 1968.   It is a relatively small department since many of its functions were hived off following the recommendations of the Fulton Report (1968). Among other things, the Fulton Report advocated the decentralisation of some departmental functions to autonomous, non-departmental agencies in order to foster accountability and free managers from bureaucratic constraints.   As a consequence, many of the Department's functions were devolved to three public bodies, the Health and Safety Commission, the Advisory Conciliation and Arbitration Service (ACAS) and the Manpower Services Commission (MSC).

The specific concerns of MAFF and the DTI for the health and welfare of the alcohol and tobacco industries are reinforced by the DoEmp, which has general oversight of, and responsibility for, employment policy. Thus, any proposals which would adversely affect employment prospects in the tobacco and allied industries or which were designed to reduce per capita alcohol consumption, such as those proposed by the national alcohol agency (Alcohol Concern, 1987), are of direct interest to the Department's Employment Policy Branch. Like the DTI, the DoEmp constantly monitors other departments for policy proposals or developments in existing policies which might have employment consequences.

Whilst the Department does not have specific responsibility for either the tobacco or alcohol industries, it is concerned with one area of economic activity which has important implications for alcohol policy. The DoEmp is the governmental sponsor for the tourist industry whose interest and concerns are the responsibility of Branch 3 in its Small Firms and Tourism (SFT) Division. This branch contains three sections. Section A deals with matters relating to the English Tourist Board whilst Section B is responsible for all matters involving the British Tourist Authority (BTA). Section C liaises with other government departments over key issues, such as the education and training of workers in the tourist industry and on liquor licensing issues.

The representations of the tourist industry have been at the forefront of the campaign to relax the liquor licensing hours in England and Wales. The English Tourist Board and the BTA are largely independent bodies although they are financed by government. They have lobbied energetically for changes to a law which they believe has adversely affected the British tourist industry. In July 1986, the BTA wrote to all MPs seeking their support for

146

changes and the SFT Division was actively involved in the inter-departmental lobbying process. SFT3's main inter-departmental link over reform was with the Home Office where a Liquor Licensing Section is located within Division A of the Criminal Justice and Constitutional Department. The Home Office has the lead responsibility in this policy area because it is seen primarily as a public order and law enforcement issue.

Because of the nature of its responsibilities, the Home Office is frequently depicted as a regulatory department where bureaucratic attention to detail sets the tone of organisational culture. However, it should be emphasised that whilst its organisational culture in respect of existing obligations may be regulatory, one of its principal and abiding aims is to resist the pressure from other parts of government to solve every problem with a fresh set of laws. This being so, demands for the lifting of legal controls are likely to be received favourably, assuming that it can be demonstrated to ministers' satisfaction that no deleterious effects will follow. The case in favour of the licensing law reform sought by the trade and supported by SFT3 in the Department of Employment was, to all intents and purposes, settled by the Office of Population Censuses and Surveys (OPCS) report commissioned by the Scottish Office to examine the impact on drinking patterns of the Licensing Act (Scotland) 1976, which relaxed aspects of the licensing law in that country (Goddard, 1986). However, the decision to press ahead with the reform owed as much to the Conservative Party's ideological commitment to deregulation, as to bureaucratic considerations.

CONCLUSION

The pattern of departmental-group links in the alcohol and tobacco policy areas conforms to the 'clientella' model which describes the close and exclusive relationships created when government departments select particular groups as the legitimate representatives of outside interests, thus restricting the range of information and advice they receive and creating a relationship of close, mutual dependence (Peters, 1978). Certainly, neither MAFF nor the DTI actively seek contact with non-industry groups (such as those concerned with the health consequences of alcohol and tobacco consumption) nor is such contact usually sought by the groups themselves. Moreover, the exclusiveness of the departmental-group links is reinforced, in the case of alcohol, by the obligations which sponsorship imposes and which institutionalises the clientella relationship. However there is nothing exceptional in this relationship as producer groups of all kinds have close links with government and their concerns are given high priority because of the sanctions they can wield and their role in the economy. Thus, impediments to the development of a coordinated prevention strategy are well entrenched in the functionally differentiated departmental structure in the British government with its associated networks and the priorities it embodies.

Given the industry's close and complex links with government, alterations to both organisational structure and process may well be necessary if coordinated prevention strategies are to be developed. Some of the departments such as the Home Office, the Department of Health and the Scottish Office have an alcohol policy coordinator because their interests are fragmented among a variety of internal administrative units. However, organisational responsibilities within the producer departments and others with alcohol and tobacco responsibilities are internally fragmented. Policy making within and between departments and across organisational networks would be facilitated if all had similar coordinators to promote communication, disseminate views, identify problems and help shape common goals. A start in this direction has been made with the establishment of the Ministerial Group on Alcohol Misuse but much more could be done to facilitate linkages between networks and expose insulated policy making processes to wider considerations.

In addition, it may be appropriate to end governmental sponsorship of the alcohol industry by moving the industry to the DTI. The MAFF is a relatively small department with a narrow range of responsibilities. Departments of this kind can more easily be 'captured' by client groups and it is sometimes alleged that the National Farmers Union has come to dominate policy making in the MAFF. Farming interests are closely entwined with those of the drinks industry and transferring the latter to the DTI might have practical as well as symbolic importance. The effect of the DTI's decision to end sponsorship on the Department's relationships with groups is unclear and it may have the effect of strengthening the industries which it intends should be more self-reliant. However, the policy is intended to take into account the interests of consumers, in a way which was not done when the Department simply provided industries with a voice in government. Clearly, the interests of consumers could and should involve a consideration of the health consequences of industrial and employment policies. Moreover, the DTI has an important cluster of alcohol concerns including consumer safety, weights and measures and sickness and absenteeism. If it were to take over responsibility for the alcohol industry it would be in a position to coordinate production and consumption issues.

The impediments to a coordinated prevention strategy though well embedded, are not immovable. A number of initiatives could be promoted to expose the departments at the heart of the producer networks to other considerations and influences and to better inform the policy process. Consideration could be given as to whether the alcohol industry should be sponsored and to which department it should be linked. In addition, it must be recognised that the power and strength of the alcohol and tobacco producers rest not just on their institutional links and relationships with government but on their own claims to economic indispensability. Appropriate changes to governmental structures and processes will be difficult as long as these are taken at face value. Thus, the succeeding chapters look in detail at the economic and employment characteristics of the industries and examine the possible impact which prevention policy might have on them.

References

Alcohol Concern, (1987), *The Drinking Revolution*, Alcohol Concern, London.

Ashford, D.E., (1981), *Policy and Politics in Britain*, Basil Blackwell, Oxford.

Beer, S.H., (1965), *Modern British Politics*, Faber and Faber, London.

Booth, M., Hardman, G. and Hartley, K., (1986), 'Data Note 6, The UK alcohol and tobacco industries', *British Journal of Addiction*, 81, 825-830.

Burch, M., (1987), 'The demise of cabinet Government', in Robins, L., (ed.), *Political Institutions in Britain: Development and Change*, Longman, London and New York.

Cabinet Office, (1985), *Lifting the Burden*, Cmnd. 9571, HMSO, London.

Central Policy Review Staff (CPRS), (1979), *Alcohol Policies*, Reprinted (1982), University of Stockholm, Stockholm.

Department of Employment (DoEmp), (1986), *Building Businesses ... Not Barriers*, Cmnd. 9794, HMSO, London.

Downs, A., (1957), *An Economic Theory of Democracy*, Harper and Row, New York.

Friend, J., Power, J. and Yewlett, C., (1974), *Public Planning: the inter-corporate dimension*, Tavistock, London.

Fulton Report, (1986), *The Civil Service, Vol.1: Report of the Committee*, Cmnd. 3638, HMSO, London.

Goddard, E., (1986), *Drinking and Attitudes to Licensing in Scotland*, Office of Population, Censures and Surveys (OPCS), HMSO, London.

Greenwood, J. and Wilson, D., (1984), *Public Administration in Britain*, George Allen and Unwin, London.

Griffith, J.A.G., (1966), *Central Departments and Local Authorities*, Allen and Unwin, London.

Haldane Report, (1918), *Report of the Machinery of Government Committee*, Cmnd. 9230, HMSO, London.

Ham, C., (1982), *Health Policy in Britain*, Macmillan, London.

Harrison, L. and Tether, P., (1987), 'The coordination of UK policy on alcohol and tobacco: the significance of organisational networks', *Policy and Politics*, (15) 2, 77-90.

Heclo, H. and Wildavsky, A., (1981), *The Private Government of Public Money*, Macmillan, London.

Hjern, B. and Porter, D., (1981), 'Implementation structures, a new unit of administrative analysis', *Organisation Studies*, (2), 3, 211-227.

Home Office, (1987), *News Release*, September 18, London.

Home Office, (1987), Standing Conference on Crime Prevention Working Group, *Young People and Alcohol*, Home Office, London.

Jennings, I., (1959), *The Law and the Constitution*, 5th ed., University of London Press, London.

Ministry of Agriculture, Fisheries and Food (MAFF), (1987), *Strength of Alcoholic Drinks to be Declared*, Press Release 246/87, London.

Norton, P., (1987), 'Parliament and policy in Britain: the House of Commons as a policy influencer', in Robins, L. (ed.), *Topics in British Politics 2*, Political Education Press, London.

Peters, G., (1978), *The Politics of Bureaucracy*, Longman, New York and London.

Privy Council, (1988), *New Measures to Tackle Alcohol Abuse*, Press Release, January 18, London.

Richardson, J. and Jordan, G., (1979), *Governing Under Pressure*, Martin Robertson, Oxford.

Saunders, P., (1981), *Social Theory and the Urban Question*, Hutchinson, London.

Stanyer, J., and Smith, B., (1976), *Administering Britain*, Fontana/Collins, London.

Sunday Telegraph, (1988), 27 January, 4.

Sunday Times, (1973), 10 June, 10.

Sunday Times, (1988), 12 January, 8.

Waterman, M.J., (ed.), (1987), *Advertising Statistics Yearbook 1987*, The Advertising Association, London.

Williams, S., (1980), 'The decision makers', in *Policy and Practice: The Experience of Government*, RIPA, London.

8 Industry: structure, performance and policy

MARK BOOTH, KEITH HARTLEY AND MELANIE POWELL

The markets for alcohol and tobacco products reflect both demand and supply. Consumers determine demand on the basis of product prices, the prices of substitutes and incomes, together with their tastes and preferences (see Chapter 2). Groups of firms comprising industries form the supply side of the market, and they will offer alcohol and tobacco products so long as their activities are expected to be relatively profitable. In the analysis of prevention policies, much of the debate has focused on demand and consumption to the neglect of the supply side[1].

Advocates of public policies to reduce smoking and drinking cannot ignore the implications for firms supplying these products or the likely responses by firms to measures designed to reduce domestic sales. The supplying groups likely to lose from prevention policies include the managers, workers and shareholders in the UK alcohol and tobacco industries, suppliers of materials, equipment and services, and those in distribution networks including advertising agencies and retail outlets (e.g. clubs, shops, supermarkets and public houses). When new prevention measures are expected or are introduced, various interest groups representing the industry will lobby the government to modify its restrictive policies. Producers will stress the adverse effects on jobs, exports and profitability, all of which will be alleged to mean a further decline in the UK's manufacturing base. Whilst seeking to reduce the level of any tax increases or modify regulatory constraints, firms will also pursue measures to minimise the effects of these policies on themselves. For example, in response to higher taxes, firms might restrict price increases to those products where demand is relatively unresponsive to higher prices; or, they might shift the burden to part-time and unorganised workers, rather than to UK consumers and the firms' shareholders. Over time, firms can respond to actual or expected government prevention policies by introducing new products (e.g. alcohol-free drinks; safer cigarettes) and by mergers and take-overs either within the same industry or by diversifying into other markets. Policy-makers need to know how firms are likely to respond to various prevention measures. It needs to be recognised that responses by firms can be complex and might occur over a long period of time and some responses might be viewed as socially undesirable.

This chapter provides an overview of the UK alcohol and tobacco industries. It describes their size, structure and performance. Attention is given to mergers, diversification and profitability. Questions arise as to whether mergers and diversification are possible responses to actual and potential government prevention measures; whether acquisitions have created large producer interest groups able to influence the taxation and regulatory policies of vote-sensitive governments; and whether mergers have resulted in monopolies which might act against the public interest. Claims by the industries that taxation and other prevention policies have had an adverse effect on profitability need to be tested. Also, the experience of the UK tobacco industry might provide insights into the future response of the alcohol industry to possible new prevention policies reflecting growing public concern over the health and public order aspects of alcohol consumption. Detailed studies of the Scotch whisky industry and of the employment effects of prevention policies are presented in Chapters 9 and 10. Throughout this chapter, the aim is to show that a study of the supply side is an important component of the overall market for alcohol and tobacco products and cannot be ignored in debates about prevention policy.

THE ALCOHOL AND TOBACCO INDUSTRIES

A framework for analysing the industry

Any industry can be analysed by using a structure-performance framework. This traditional approach stresses that the performance of an industry depends on its structure. Industry performance is measured by labour productivity, exports, profitability and, ultimately, efficiency, whilst structure is reflected in the number of firms, their size and entry conditions. Two polar market situations are contrasted, namely, the economic models of perfect competition and monopoly. Perfect competition is characterised by large numbers of small firms and free entry into the industry resulting in an efficient market solution. By comparison, monopoly consists of a single seller with no close substitutes, resulting in higher prices, lower output, continued excessive profits, and an inefficient use of resources, all of which have been criticised as socially undesirable (Scherer, 1980). Between the polar extremes of monopoly and perfect competition, there are a variety of intermediate industry structures such as oligopoly which comprises a small number of large firms. In oligopoly industries, firms compete through a variety of non-price activities, such as advertising, marketing and product differentiation (e.g. brands), any of which may lead to the excesses and wastes associated with inefficiency. Where there are very few firms, there is the possibility of collusion either implicitly or explicitly through cartels or restrictive practices designed to achieve monopoly outcomes. Some of the general features of oligopolies are characteristics of the UK alcohol and tobacco industries.

The traditional structure-performance framework predicts that firms with monopoly power will be associated with continued high profits and inefficiency. The degree of monopoly power possessed by a firm can be measured by the concentration ratio which shows the proportion of industry output produced by the largest firm or by, say, the top five firms. However, the structure-performance framework has been subject to a variety of criticisms. It is assumed that firms are profit-maximisers, but, where markets are not perfectly competitive, firms might pursue other objectives such as sales, growth or managerial satisfaction. In addition, it is recognised that mergers and monopolies might offer compensating benefits in the form of research and development leading to technical progress and the economies of large-scale operations; factors which might be regarded as socially acceptable and in the public interest. Some critics reject the static structure-performance framework and stress the creative role of the entrepreneur in a world of ignorance and uncertainty. If markets are dynamic, competition is a continuous process and monopoly is only a temporary phenomenon which will attract profit-seeking rivals (Kirzner, 1973). A more recent development stresses contestability, claiming that the threat of entry will force existing firms in an industry to behave competitively.

Any one of the models identified above could be used by government to predict the supply side effects of its prevention policies and to determine whether such effects are sociably desirable. Government analysts must choose a theory of firm behaviour and of market structure to explain observed responses by the UK alcohol and tobacco industries. In the circumstances, the structure-performance framework provides a useful taxonomy and a starting point for analysing the industries; but alternative models need to be applied to determine whether they offer different insights and predictions. In all cases, firms are central to any analysis of the industry and prevention policy.

Industrial responses to prevention policies

In formulating prevention policies, it should not be assumed that firms will be passive organisations. Instead, firms can be viewed as active and adaptable agents who may respond to new prevention policies by seeking alternative ways of improving performance in situations characterised by ignorance and uncertainty about market opportunities. Firms can be compared with a balloon : no sooner is one part squeezed, then another part expands! Thus, a tax on a firm's products need not be shifted forward to consumers in higher prices. Instead, the tax might be shifted backwards to the factors of production in the form of labour, shareholders, or the suppliers of equipment and materials either in the UK or overseas. Similarly, firms can respond to an actual or expected reduction in their domestic sales by greater advertising or marketing efforts, by increasing exports of their existing products, by introducing new products, by acquiring rivals at home or overseas or by diversifying into completely new product markets in the UK or abroad. The success of these various reactions by firms will determine profitability and their willingness to remain in the alcohol and tobacco markets. Because of the diversity of reactions by firms and the time-period over which adjustments occur, the analysis of the supply side and market effects of prevention policies can be extremely complex.

Depending on policy circumstances, firms are likely to adopt different methods of improving performance. Some might choose to specialise (e.g. brewers), whilst others will diversify but into different markets (e.g. cigarette companies). Even in a specialist market such as brewing, firms can adopt different solutions. For example, unlike the other major brewers, Guinness has never owned its retail outlets. These variations may arise because those who control company policy hold different views about the prospects for profits. The relative importance of transactions costs of organising vertically-integrated firms with tied outlets compared with relying upon external market transactions may also be an explanatory factor. Entrepreneurs have to bear the risks and consequences of discovering profitable opportunities before their rivals. Those who guess correctly will survive and those who make mistakes will fail. Ultimately, shareholders will continue to invest in alcohol and tobacco production for as long as these are perceived to be worthwhile and funds will be withdrawn when other markets offer more attractive prospects.

When faced with prevention measures which might affect adversely their profitability, firms may also resort to lobbying activities in order to persuade vote-conscious governments to modify such policies. Large firms and trade associations representing the interest of groups such as the brewers, the Scotch whisky industry and tobacco retailers (see Chapter 5), will lobby government if the outcome is perceived to be worthwhile. These interest groups appear to be well-informed in their specialist areas. They can speak with experience about the likely effects of prevention policies on their companies, on jobs, on exports and on the local economy; they can support their arguments with consultancy reports prepared by experts and they can hire public relations firms to disseminate the evidence to politicians and to the wider community. From an industrial perspective, successful lobbying might be reflected in relatively low tax increases, exemptions from higher taxes (e.g. to provide exports), the introduction of voluntary self-regulation rather than compulsory legislation (e.g. advertising), or subsequent modifications in the implementation of a penal policy. For the purpose of this chapter, it is sufficient to recognise that the alcohol and tobacco industries will seek to prevent or modify policies which might have an adverse effect on their business. In this context, it has been suggested that the alcohol and tobacco industries comprise powerful producer groups which have been successful in influencing government policy in their favour. If so, a study of these industries and of their constituent companies could provide insights into the characteristics of powerful producer groups. A starting point is the definition of the industry.

Defining the industry

Any prevention policy involving suppliers has to start from a clear definition of the relevant industry. Unfortunately for policy-makers, industries are not homogeneous entities consisting of a group of firms producing identical products. Instead, an industry can be defined as a group of firms producing similar products, with boundaries determined by a gap in the chain of substitutes. Problems arise in identifying similar products and substitutes, and in determining the magnitude of the gap required in the chain of substitutes. From a consumer's viewpoint, there are numerous products from UK and foreign firms, many of which they regard as substitutes. Cigarettes and beer might be partial substitutes as might other addictive products such as heroin, some foods and even jogging. This highlights the problem facing any government seeking to reduce the consumption of one addictive substance such as tobacco; consumers will always search for alternative ways of meeting their demands and profit-seeking firms will respond either legally or illegally (via black markets).

155

The UK alcohol and tobacco industries comprise privately-owned domestic manufacturers involved in supplying home and export markets in competition with European and other foreign firms. Inevitably, defining an industry requires arbitrary judgements. The Government's Standard Industrial Classification (SIC) defines the tobacco industry as manufacturing tobacco, cigars, cigarettes and snuff (SIC 429). In contrast, the UK alcohol industry is not a single entity but consists of a number of sectors, namely brewing and malting (SIC 427), spirit distilling and compounding (SIC 424) and wines, cider and perry (SIC 426). In addition, as a further substitute, there is a UK soft drinks industry which manufactures mineral waters, soft drinks, fruit and vegetable juices (SIC 428). Evidence on the size of the UK alcohol and tobacco industries is shown in Table 8.1. The emphasis on UK manufacturers excludes the distribution sector which is especially important for the brewing industry in relation to tied houses.

The brewing and tobacco companies dominate the UK alcohol and tobacco industries output and employment. Together, they account for almost 5 per cent of the gross output of UK manufacturing industry and 2.5 per cent of its net output. Interestingly, in both 1975 and 1985, labour productivity in the alcohol and tobacco industries considerably exceeded the average for UK manufacturing. Table 8.1 can also be used to show the changing shares of output by different sections in the UK alcohol, drinks and tobacco industries as a group. Between 1975 and 1986, the UK wines and spirits sectors increased their share of the group's total net output, whilst the brewers and tobacco companies experienced a decline in share.

Analysis of the industry is further complicated because some of the sectors can be sub-divided into specialist product groups each with their distinctive characteristics. The tobacco companies produce cigars, pipe tobacco and a range of cigarette brands segmented by size, tar content and price. The brewers produce various types of beers and lagers in both draught and packaged forms, whilst the spirits industry is sub-divided into gin, vodka, whisky and other drinks produced in the UK or imported. Wines, most of which are imported into the UK, can be separated from cider and perry. Some companies are involved in more than one sector of an industry, in particular the major brewers control a substantial part of the wines and spirits markets. There are also examples of firms which have been involved in both tobacco and alcohol. In the tobacco industry, Rothmans owns brewery operations in Canada and Eire, and until 1986, Imperial also had a brewery division (Courage). Moreover, some companies have diversified outside their traditional industry boundaries, making the comparisons of data published at the industry level (SIC) with that provided in a company's annual reports more difficult. The tobacco companies, for example, are also involved in engineering, financial services, office products and retailing. Questions

Table 8.1
The UK alcohol and tobacco industries

	1975	1985	1986
1. Gross output (£m)[b]			
Brewing & malting	1950.6	4748.0	4995.7
Spirit distilling	989.9	2077.5	2188.2
Wines, cider & perry	103.9	424.7	438.8
Soft drinks	543.5	1315.9	1639.9
Tobacco	2476.1	5770.3	5684.4
UK manufacturing	93048.0	226636.0	(n/a)
2. Net output (£m)[a,b]			
Brewing & malting	613.3	1240.6	1375.1
Spirit distilling	297.8	888.5	872.5
Wines, cider & perry	46.3	160.1	176.5
Soft drinks	233.3	449.9	563.0
Tobacco	397.5	1137.0	935.8
UK manufacturing	36948.0	94385.1	(n/a)
3. Employment (000's)			
Brewing & malting	66.2	35.6	35.3
Spirit distilling	26.0	16.4	16.1
Wines, cider & perry	5.1	4.3	4.1
Soft drinks	27.9	17.4	18.9
Tobacco	39.8	23.9	20.5
4. Net output per head (£)[a,b]			
Brewing & malting	9261	34816	39010
Spirit distilling	11451	54222	54198
Wines, cider & perry	9068	37586	42664
Soft drinks	8370	25882	29809
Tobacco	9981	47629	45613
UK manufacturing	4948	18969	(n/a)
5. Retail price index (15th Jan. 1974 = 100)			
Alcoholic drink	135.2	412.1	430.6
Tobacco	147.7	532.5	584.9

a. Net output is gross output minus purchases of materials and goods, stock changes and excise payments.

b. Value figures are in current prices.

Sources: Business Monitor, *Report on the Census of Production,* Industry Reports and Summary Tables, HMSO, London, 1976, 1985 and 1986; *Monthly Digest of Statistics,* HMSO, London, 1986.

157

arise as to whether company involvement in different sub-sectors within or across industry results from changing market opportunities at home and overseas, alone, or also results from actual and expected prevention policies.

Supply side markets trends

Data on the value of output for the UK alcohol and tobacco industries for the period 1963-86 are shown in Table 8.2. The value figures reflect changes in quality and they have been deflated to remove the effects of inflation. For recent years, the general picture shows a declining output for the major industrial sectors. The output of the UK tobacco industry has declined substantially and by 1986 was slightly more than 50 per cent of its 1973 peak. Several factors may account for this major reduction, including the effects of recession and unemployment in the UK, the effects of taxation, advertising controls, health education campaigns and competition from foreign suppliers. Some simple correlations between the dates of policy changes and trends in the industry's output are suggestive. In the context of health education as part of prevention policy, it is significant that the Royal College of Physicians published its first report on the health effects of smoking in 1962, followed by a second report in 1971. In 1965, there was a TV ban on cigarette advertising and voluntary health warnings on cigarette packets were introduced in 1971. However, the long-run decline in the industry's sales started after 1973 and coincided with a succession of prevention measures concerned with advertising controls, health warnings, tax increases and further reports on health and smoking from the Royal College of Physicians.

Evidence from company reports suggests that the tobacco industry perceive higher taxation to be the major cause of declining domestic sales. Changes in the excise tax rate on cigarettes substantially exceeded the rate of inflation in 1974, 1975, 1977, 1981, 1984 and 1986 (see Chapter 5). There are, however, other influences on the industry's domestic sales such as increased competition from imports and the general recession during the 1970s and into the 1980s when UK unemployment rates rose from 2.4 per cent in 1973 to some 14 per cent in 1986. It must also be remembered that the total output figures for the UK tobacco industry include exports so that explanations of changing sales have to include an analysis of both the home and overseas markets, including the competitiveness of British and foreign firms. Faced with prospects of declining domestic sales, UK firms are likely to seek alternative markets overseas (Cooper, Hartley and Harvey, 1970). In fact, the UK tobacco industry increased the proportion of its output for export from some 3 per cent in 1973 to 8 per cent in 1986. However, overseas markets have also been subject to recession, higher taxation on tobacco products and the development of local manufacturing operations, all of which have adversely affected UK exports and contributed further to the decline in total output. In the circumstances, the UK tobacco industry has every inducement to attribute all its problems to the British Government's taxation policy. At the same time, faced with a declining trend in output, profit-conscious firms will seek alternative market opportunities. As a result of acquisitions, the UK tobacco companies have become large diversified groups with an extensive and varied range of other products, all of which offers some protection from the immediate impact of anti-smoking campaigns (see below).

For the UK brewers and distillers, output peaked in the late 1970s after which it showed a declining trend. By 1986, output of the UK brewing industry was 70 per cent of its 1979 level, whilst spirits production showed some recovery after 1984. In contrast, the output of the relatively small British wines, cider and perry sector showed a long-run rising trend, reflecting changing tastes and substitution effects in the UK alcohol market. Since most wines are imported into the UK (over 90 per cent), such changes are more accurately reflected in consumer expenditure patterns. In 1963, wines, cider and perry accounted for some 11 per cent of UK consumer expenditure on alcoholic drinks, with beer accounting for 67 per cent and spirits 22 per cent. By 1986, the corresponding figures were 26 per cent for wines, 48 per cent for beers and 26 per cent for spirits (see Chapter 1, Table 1.1). Fiscal policy can obviously influence consumption patterns by changing relative prices. Changes in excise tax rates which considerably exceeded the rate of inflation occurred for beers and wines in 1974, for beers, wines and spirits in 1975 and 1981, and for beer in 1984. However, spirits usually received a relatively favourable tax treatment. Moreover, in some years, such as 1977-79 and 1986, changes in excise duties on alcohol were substantially below the rate of inflation (Chapter 5).

The broad changes in the UK alcohol market conceal further developments in the different product groups. Within the beer market, the market share for lagers increased from 24 per cent in 1976 to some 43 per cent in 1986. During the same period, the market share of canned beers to all beer sales increased from 7 per cent to 15 per cent. The share of imported beers in total UK consumption also increased from 4.6 per cent in 1976 to 6.3 per cent in 1986 (Brewers Society, 1988). Imported beers are produced mainly in Ireland (Guinness), West Germany and the Netherlands. However, between 1976 and 1986, the beer import market changed substantially, with West Germany, the Netherlands and Australia accounting for a larger share of imports, whilst Ireland and Denmark experienced a substantial decline in market share. However, import figures for beer do not represent the proportion of foreign beers consumed in the UK market. Foreign suppliers tend to expand into the UK market by import penetration initially and then switch to licensed production to reduce transport costs. For example, Allied Lyons has licences to produce Castlemaine, Skol, Lowenbrau and Orangebaum, whilst Grand Metropolitan brews Budweiser, Carlsberg and Fosters under licence in the UK.

Table 8.2

Output of UK alcohol and tobacco industries

(£m 1980 prices)

Year	Brewing[a] and malting	Spirit distilling[c] and rectifying	British[c] wines cider & perry	Tobacco[b]
1963	2993.4	985.8	67.4	4550.2
1968	3372.5	1278.7	89.1	4284.3
1970	3402.5	1662.2	124.1	4487.4
1971	3559.6	1664.1	140.1	4392.0
1972	3358.9	1549.8	130.7	4466.5
1973	3902.2	1741.0	149.0	5159.5
1974	3758.7	2062.1	166.1	4914.9
1975	3659.7	1677.9	176.3	4671.9
1976	3781.0	1891.4	168.2	4682.6
1977	3736.8	1783.4	186.3	4274.8
1978	3941.1	2153.6	198.9	4401.6
1979	3963.0	2264.8	222.2	3816.5
1980	3523.6	1924.0	208.0	4159.2
1981	3262.3	1633.9	220.5	3636.9
1982	2946.4	1567.7	231.0	3528.9
1983	2979.4	1523.8	233.5	3469.8
1984	2858.7	1471.7	270.7	3321.0
1985	2722.5	1486.1	303.8	3054.7
1986	2728.4	1522.8	305.4	2723.7

a. Brewing and malting figures deflated by Producer Price Index for beer.
b. Tobacco figures deflated by Producer Price Index for tobacco.
c. Spirit figures and BWC and P figures deflated by Retail Price index for wines and spirits. 1980 prices.

Source: Census of production, Business Statistics Office, HMSO (annual).

A further development is the increasingly international and global nature of the drinks industry. UK brewers have created overseas subsidiaries, acquired foreign firms and have entered into international partnership agreements. For example, Grand Metropolitan's International Distillers and Vintners subsidiary is one of the world's leading wines and spirits companies, whilst Guinness is a joint owner of Louis Vuitton Moet Hennessy (LVMH) the French cognac company. Similarly, the Australian companies of Bond (Castlemaine) and Elders IXL (Fosters) have acquired interests in breweries in Canada, the USA and the UK (Elders acquired Courage); and the Canadian Seagram company acquired the French cognac firm of Martell. These changes in ownership indicate the extent of response to changing market opportunities and suggest the need for an analysis of companies. A company analysis could also identify the characteristics of firms as producer groups in opposition to prevention policies.

THE COMPANIES

Explaining the size of firms

The major alcohol and tobacco companies are amongst the largest enterprises in the UK, with seven companies in the top 50 in 1987 (Table 8.3). The tobacco companies are all large, diversified enterprises with a wide range of other activities such as engineering, financial services, luxury consumer products, paper manufacturing and printing. The large national brewers have tied outlets (except for Guinness), are diversified into related markets, especially wines and spirits, and operate on an international scale. There are also smaller firms in the alcohol industry mostly specialising as regional brewers or distillers (Booth et al., 1988).

The current size of firms and resulting structure of the UK alcohol and tobacco industries reflects the growth of companies through either internal expansion or mergers and take-overs. The choice between these alternative methods of growth will depend on their relative costs and profitability. By increasing their size, firms can obtain any available economies of large-scale operations and may also acquire a degree of monopoly power, potentially increasing profitability. Economies of scale are an important determinant of firm size and industry structure. Where scale economies are substantial, the UK market might only be able to support one or a relatively small number of firms so that there will be a conflict between firms of efficient scale and competition. In such cases, efficient scale might imply a domestic monopoly, with possible adverse effects on prices, output, efficiency and dynamism.

Size and unit costs

Only limited evidence is available on economies of scale, especially for tobacco, and much of the evidence is dated. An early 1970s estimate suggested that for the tobacco companies, most of the available economies

161

of large-scale operations are obtained at an annual output of 36 billion cigarettes equivalent to 21 per cent of UK output in 1973 (Cmnd. 7198, 1978, p.87; Scherer 1973). Such scale factors are one explanation of the relatively small number of tobacco companies in the domestic market. In fact, the tobacco industry is one of the most highly concentrated industries in the UK, with a five-firm concentration ratio for output of 99 per cent (Table 8.4). Other UK manufacturing industries with a five-firm concentration ratio of 80 per cent or more in 1985 included ordnance and small arms, motor vehicles, man-made fibres, cement and the extraction and preparation of metal ores. An extremely high level of concentration has been a feature of the tobacco industry throughout the century. In 1984, four multinational corporations dominated the UK tobacco industry. These were Imperial (now a subsidiary of Hanson Trust) with a 44 per cent share, Gallaher (a subsidiary of American Brands) with a 32 per cent share, Rothmans International with a 15 per cent share, and British American Tobacco (BAT) industries, a British firm and the world's largest tobacco company, which concentrates on overseas sales.

Scale economies are believed to be substantial in the brewing industry and are one of the factors contributing to the mergers of the 1960s. Estimates for brewing suggest a minimum efficient scale (mes) of plant of 1m to 1.8m barrels per annum, equivalent to 3 per cent to 4.5 per cent of the UK market; but other studies in the 1970s have estimated mes plants of as little as 1 per cent and as high as 13 per cent of the UK market (Brouwer, 1981; Cockerill, 1977; Cmnd. 7198, 1978, p.87; Rees, 1973; Scherer, 1973). An increase in the annual output of beer from 0.6m to 1.8m barrels could reduce unit costs by almost 15 per cent (excluding taxes: Cockerill, 1977, p.289). However, whilst there are economies from a larger output associated with supplying a national market, it is also noticeable that a number of smaller brewers have survived by specialising in local or regional beers (real ale). As a result, the UK brewing industry is dominated by seven major national brewers and a number of smaller local breweries, giving a five-firm concentration ratio of 50 per cent for gross output in 1985 (Table 8.4). Other UK manufacturing industries with a similar five-firm concentration ratio in 1985 included basic electrical equipment, basic industrial chemicals, office machinery and telecommunications. The major UK brewers are Allied-Lyons, Bass, Courage (Elders), Grand Metropolitan, Guinness, Scottish and Newcastle and Whitbread. In the early 1980s, Bass had the largest share of the UK market with 20 per cent, followed by Allied with a 14 per cent market share (Booth et al., 1986).

Table 8.3
UK alcohol and tobacco companies

Company	UK ranking by sales	Turnover (£m)	Employment	Profit rate[a] (%)	Main activity
BAT Industries	3	13623	176370	22.3	Tobacco, financial services, retailing, paper, packaging.
Grand Metro-politan	13	5291.3	131493	14.6	Hotels, consumer services, food, brewers, wines & spirits.
Hanson Trust (Imperial)	17	4312	92000	13.9	Industrial services, building products, food products, tobacco.
Allied-Lyons	23	3614.8	77549	16.8	Brewers, wines, spirits, food, hotels.
Gallaher	26	3404.7	30328	27.0	Tobacco, optical, pumps and valves, houseware.
Bass	37	2709.7	76922	19.7	Brewers, soft drinks, wines and spirits merchants, hotels, holidays.
Guinness	39	2601.6	32062	14.6	Brewers, distillers, retailing, publishing.
Whitbread	73	1553.9	47723	12.4	Brewers, wines, spirits, restaurants.
Rothmans	76	1446.9	21833	15.9	Tobacco, luxury consumer products.
Scottish and Newcastle	137	773.6	20361	16.6	Brewers, wines, spirits, hotels.

a.   Profit are net profits before interest and tax as a return on capital.

Sources: *Times 1000, 1987–88,* Times Books, London; Company Reports.

Table 8.4

Concentration in UK alcohol and tobacco industries

| Year | 5 firm concentration ratio for output | |
	Brewing (%)	Tobacco (%)
1963	51	99.7
1968	62	99.9
1971	58	99.0
1985	50	99.0

Source: Business monitor, *Report on the Census of Production,* Summary Tables, HMSO, London, 1963, 1968, 1971, 1985.

The major brewers gain some commercial advantage through owning retail outlets (tied-houses) through economies in delivery, administration and monitoring costs. The ability to monitor is important when product quality is a major competitive variable (Economists Advisory Group (EAG), 1969). The system of tied-houses allows the brewer to limit on-sale competition. However, rivalry exists in the form of alternative outlets such as clubs, hotels and off-licences (shops, supermarkets). Indeed, between 1976 and 1985, the number of licensed premises owned by the brewers declined during a period when the total number of licensed premises increased substantially. By 1985, brewery-owned licensed premises accounted for some 27 per cent of all licences compared with 36 per cent in 1976 (Brewers Society, 1986).

Whilst economies of scale are an important determinant of firm size and industry structure, they are concerned with the output of a single product. Enterprises, especially in alcohol and tobacco, are multi-product organisations and their size and scope could be explained by the benefits of diversification. A firm might diversify in order to reduce the financial risks associated with dependence on one activity. Diversification enables a firm to spread the risks of uncertainty in market operations. The UK tobacco companies are an obvious example of such risk spreading behaviour. Also, diversification might enable a firm to use more profitably its available assets in the form of plant and equipment, managers, scientists and their technical knowledge, skilled labour, marketing expertise, goodwill and established brand names (e.g. Boots, Marks and Spencer, Sainsbury). In some cases, cost savings may result from a multi-product output. Such economies of scope occur where the cost of producing two or more products in combination is less than the total cost of producing each product separately (Baumol et al., 1982). Diversification can be achieved through mergers and take-overs.

Mergers and concentration

Firms can expand and increase their profits through mergers and take-overs, and both the alcohol and tobacco industries have been extensively involved in the acquisition of other companies. Indeed, these industries have taken part in some of the largest UK mergers and take-overs such as Hanson-Imperial and Guinness-Distillers in 1986 and BAT-Eagle Star in 1983 (Scouller, 1987). Significantly, the acquisitions by the UK tobacco companies have involved diversification into completely different markets, creating large conglomerates. These diversifications may represent the UK industry's response to an actual and expected decline in cigarette smoking (Table 8.3; Booth et al., 1988). By contrast, mergers in the UK brewing industry have had a major impact on its structure.

In the 1960s, most of the mergers and take-overs in brewing were between firms in the same industry. As a result, the number of brewery companies declined from 247 in 1960 to 96 in 1970. There emerged a small number of large national breweries with a network of tied-houses. Industrial concentration increased substantially between 1958 and 1968, reflecting technical, scale and legal factors (Table 8.4). During the 1950s, breweries were able to expand beyond their traditional local markets because of technical change leading to the introduction of keg beer and national distribution networks. Economies of scale meant lower unit costs from greater production. However, legal factors in the form of the licensing system restricted the number and type of retail outlets and their opening hours, so restricting entry into new markets. Faced with these licensing restrictions, the quickest and least-cost method of expanding outlets and creating a national network was to acquire other brewers with tied-houses (vertical integration). The resulting increase in concentration and its association with tied-houses raised major policy questions about monopoly and competition in the UK brewing industry during the 1960s' merger boom.

After 1968, concentration in brewing declined, partly due to the re-emergence of small local breweries catering for the real ale market. In the early 1970s, two significant take-overs occurred, namely the acquisition of Courage by Imperial and of Watney Mann by Grand Metropolitan Hotels. These acquisitions meant that two of Britain's largest brewers were now subsidiaries of non-brewing companies, one of which was a tobacco firm. The major brewers have also diversified into closely related markets such as wines and spirits, soft drinks, hotels and restaurants. This pattern of diversification probably reflects the desire to use existing managerial and marketing knowledge and skills in response to changing consumer preferences for drinks and leisure activities (Booth et al., 1988). Of course, the success or otherwise of mergers will be determined by the performance, and especially by the profitability, of the new organisation.

INDUSTRY AND COMPANY PERFORMANCE

Productivity, exports and performance

Industry and company performance is usually measured by profitability, but labour productivity and exports can also be used as indicators of factor use, technical progress and international competitiveness. Between 1960 and the 1980s, labour productivity measured in volume terms almost doubled in the UK tobacco industry and nearly trebled in brewing; and this was a period which coincided with a long-run decline in employment in both industries (see Chapter 10). In the export sphere, beer is costly to transport so that exports form only a small part of total sales. However, since 1970, the tobacco industry has increased substantially the proportion of exports in total sales, from 2.4 per cent in 1970 to some 9 per cent in the early 1980s.

A survey of 1984 data on 27 brewers and four tobacco companies, accounting for almost the total sales in each industry, provides further evidence on performance. The characteristics of the sample are summarised in Table 8.5. The averages conceal major differences with companies varying in size from under 200 to over 200,000 employees. It can be seen that the tobacco companies are larger, more diversified, have a higher labour productivity and were more profitable than the brewers. However, the differences are reduced considerably if the comparisons are made between the tobacco companies and the top five brewers. Within the brewing group, it is apparent that the larger, more diversified companies had a higher labour productivity and were more profitable than the smaller specialist brewers. Interestingly, the top five brewers appear more diversified than the tobacco companies; but usually they have diversified into the closely related food and drinks market. In contrast, the tobacco companies have diversified into completely different markets resulting in the creation of major conglomerates.

Company ownership and performance

Ownership is a major factor in determining the performance of an enterprise. Ownership patterns may reveal information about the agents who control the firm and who determine reactions to government prevention policies. Table 8.5 shows data on the average shareholding of the largest single shareholder. Not surprisingly, the smaller specialist brewers have a higher percentage of their shares held by one person or institution. In contrast, the top five brewers and the two largest tobacco companies (BAT and Imperial) had a highly dispersed share-ownership with no individual or institution owning over 6 per cent of shares. Such data might be used as an indicator of the degree to which a firm is controlled by its owners or its managers. Owner-controlled firms are more likely to be profit-seekers whereas manager controlled firms might be more concerned with sales or growth or satisfying their managers.

Table 8.5

A comparison of brewing and tobacco companies[a]

	Brewing companies		Tobacco companies	Brewing[c] and tobacco companies combined
	All	Top 5[b]		
Average size of firm				
Turnover (£m, 1984 prices)	498	2411	6119	1216
Employment	11698	56325	89103	21686
Average labour productivity (value-added, £s, 1984 prices)	9577.4	11521.4	15497.1	10341.3
Average shareholding of largest named shareholder (%)	20.9	4.6	35.4	22.8
Average profitability (return on capital: %)	12.4	19.7	27.0	14.3
Diversified brewers (n=9; %)[d]	17.3			
Specialist brewers (n=18; %)	9.9			
Average percentage of turnover outside main activity (%)	16.8	54.2	39.2	19.7
Average percentage of employment outside main activity (%)	16.4	52.5	44.3	19.9
Average percentage of turnover earned overseas (%)	3.9	19.2	36.9	8.1
Exporting breweries only (n=8; %)	13.0			

a.   Data are for 1984.

b.   Top 5 brewers are Bass, Allied Lyons, Grand Metropolitan (Watneys), Scottish and Newcastle and Whitbread. Remaining brewers are local companies.

c.   Sample: brewing n=27; tobacco n=4 (BAT, Imperial, Gallahers, and Rothmans).

d.   Diversification is measured by percentage of turnover and employment outside main activity.

Source: Company Reports.

A limited study was undertaken of share ownership in a number of brewing, distilling and tobacco companies. The exercise was explanatory and designed to illustrate the potential of the approach. In evaluating ownership and control, the focus was on ordinary shareholders who are the risk-takers and who possess full voting rights over company decisions such as the appointment of the chairman and the board of directors. Difficulties arise in determining the number of shareholders and their holdings required to exercise control over a company. A simple case is where one shareholder has a majority of shares, or where two shareholders each with more than a 25 per cent holding agree to combine their votes. However, it might not be necessary for a controlling interest to be as high as 50 per cent or more. Much depends on the size and dispersion of a company's share issue and the costs and benefits of forming a voting coalition between shareholders. It has been suggested that the proportion of shareholders required for control will vary negatively with the size and dispersion of the company's share issue (Cubbin and Leach, 1983).

In our limited study, the arbitrary decision was made to concentrate on the shares held by the top ten shareholders and the results are shown in Table 8.6. It can be seen that ownership is most highly concentrated in Whitbread and most dispersed in BAT industries. Interestingly, amongst the top 10 shareholders shown in Table 8.6, were a number of major institutional holders. These included the Prudential, the Norwich Union, the NCB Pension Fund, Legal and General and Eagle Star (acquired by BAT in 1983). In searching for the real controllers of a company, it has been argued that attention should focus on directors and inter-locking directorships. For the companies shown in Table 8.6, directors' shareholdings were usually very small, with two exceptions, namely, Whitbread and Guinness where there were substantial family shareholdings and representation on the boards of directors. This approach is useful in identifying whether companies are likely to be controlled by their shareholders or by their managers. It also identifies the major groups of individuals, families and institutions likely to lose from prevention policies. Such groups might find it worthwhile to lobby governments to modify penal policies. However, lobbying can occur through a set of informal linkages and networks, about which little is known. Alternatively, of course, shareholders can always adjust to actual or expected prevention policies through market trading as reflected in their willingness to buy and sell at a price. Much will depend on industry and company profitability.

Table 8.6

The concentration of ownership in the major UK alcohol and tobacco companies in 1984

	Top ten[a]		Top five[b]	
	%	Ranking	%	Ranking
Whitbread & Co PLC	73.9	1	69.6	1
Amalgamated Distilled Products PLC	33.6	2	26.8	2
Highland Distillers Co PLC	28.5	3	20.8	4
A Guinness and Sons PLC	28.1	4	24.2	3
Bass PLC	15.2	5	9.7	9
Scottish & Newcastle PLC	15.0	6	10.5	6
The Distillers Co PLC	14.9	7	10.8	5
Allied-Lyons PLC	13.3	8	9.7	8
Grand Metropolitan PLC	12.6	9	8.6	10
Imperial Group PLC	12.4	10	10.2	7
BAT Industries PLC	9.4	11	6.6	11

a.   Top 10 = the proportion of ordinary shares held by the top ten named shareholders.
b.   Top 5 = the proportion of ordinary shares held by the top five named shareholders.

Source: Companies House, London, Edinburgh and Cardiff.

Industrial profitability and performance

Profitability is the major indicator of industry performance. Continuously high or excessive profits could reflect monopoly power whereas repeated losses would signal the need for some adjustment in either efficiency or in the size of the industry. The profitability records of UK brewing, distilling and tobacco for 1970-83, measured as a rate of return on capital, are shown in Table 8.7. The all-industrial group provides a national average benchmark for comparative purposes. For brewing and distilling there is no indication of the continued above average or excessive profits likely to be associated with the presence and exercise of monopoly power. Profitability was below that for tobacco and usually less than the industrial average. Indeed, since 1968 concentration in brewing has declined (Table 8.4).

169

Table 8.7
Industry profitability

Year	Rate of return on capital (%) Brewers & distillers		Tobacco		All industrial groups
1970	14	(0)	17	(+3)	14
1971	15	(0)	17	(+2)	15
1972	15	(−1)	16	(0)	16
1973	15	(−3)	18	(0)	18
1974	13	(−4)	17	(0)	17
1975	13	(−3)	17	(+1)	16
1976	15	(−3)	18	(0)	18
1977	16	(−2)	18	(0)	18
1978	16	(−1)	18	(+1)	17
1979	15	(−1)	20	(+4)	16
1980	13	(−1)	18	(+4)	14
1981	13	(−1)	21	(+7)	14
1982	14	(0)	21	(+7)	14
1983	15	(0)	22	(+7)	15

Figures in brackets show the difference between the industry sector and the all industrial groups.

Source: *Bank of England Quarterly Bulletin*, September 1984.

Compared with brewing and distilling, tobacco's profitability has generally exceeded the industrial average. After 1978, tobacco industry profitability increased to a peak of 22 per cent in 1983 at a time when the total industrial group profits moved in the opposite direction.

Clearly, the level of concentration in the tobacco industry has remained unchanged throughout the period and so cannot explain the rise in profitability after 1978 (Table 8.4). Nonetheless, the high concentration ratio for tobacco might partly explain why its profitability exceeded the national average between 1970 and 1983. There are at least three other possible explanations. Declining domestic sales could have shocked the tobacco industry into increased efficiency (see Chapter 10); the industry may have responded to losses of domestic sales by increasing exports of cigarettes; or the industry may have responded to reduced cigarette sales by diversifying into other markets. In each case prevention policies may have affected company profitability and subsequently industry structure through diversification and merger.

170

Evaluating the impact of prevention policies on profits

Industry representatives and interest groups have claimed that increased taxation and other prevention policies such as advertising regulations have adversely affected profitability. The implication is that reduced profits would persuade investors to re-allocate resources to other sectors, leading to plant closures, job losses and reduced exports in the penalised sectors (see Chapter 10). In this context, the tobacco industry is particularly interesting. Given the repeated protests about the effects of increased levels of taxation, it might be expected that the UK tobacco industry would have a relatively poor profit record and would be characterised by exits from the industry. Yet the industry's profitability record has exceeded the national average (see Table 8.7). However, as profitability is determined by a variety of factors, a simple time-series of profits might not reflect the full impact of prevention policies.

To test for the possible effects of prevention policies on profitability, a statistical model was formulated and applied to both the brewing and tobacco industries for the period 1960-83. In the single equation model, industry profitability depended on the concentration ratio, output, exports, advertising and productivity. In addition, a set of public policy variables was included in which the impact of prevention policy was measured by taxation as reflected in the real tax yield, Health Education Council expenditures and dummy variables for health shocks, the 1964 changes in the licensing laws and the political composition of the government. There are the inevitable difficulties in all empirical work. Profits and capital are subject to the flexible definitions of accountants; for diversified firms, profitability reflects performance over a range of product groups so concealing the results for brewing and tobacco; and for the brewers, owing to the absence of data, it had to be assumed that brewing profitability could be represented by profitability in the drinks industry. Nevertheless, empirical work in this area is justified by the frequency with which the alcohol and tobacco industries have claimed that prevention policies have adversely affected profitability.

In testing the statistical model, it was expected that industry profitability would be reduced by increased taxation, Health Education Council spending, by Labour Governments and by health shocks (i.e. the various reports of the Royal College of Physicians on the dangers of smoking and the TV ban on cigarette advertising in 1965). For brewing, it was expected that the liberalisation associated with the 1964 changes in the licensing of outlets which relaxed the restrictions on the availability of alcohol would have had a once-for-all favourable effect on profitability. The results were suggestive rather than conclusive, with the model explaining over 70 per cent of the variations in profitability for both alcohol and tobacco[2].

For the brewing industry, it was found that taxation had the expected negative effect on profitability. A 1 per cent increase in the real tax yield might reduce profitability by some 0.5 per cent, suggesting the incidence effects were not confined to capital. Some relationships were unexpected. For example, the concentration ratio for brewing showed a negative relationship with profitability. This might reflect the adverse effects on profitability of the merger boom in brewing, such a finding being consistent with other studies of the effects of mergers on profits (Meeks, 1977). Elsewhere, there was no evidence of any impact of the governing party, nor of the 1964 changes in the licensing laws.

For the tobacco industry, many of the variables in the statistical model showed no significant relationship with profitability. The exceptions were exports which were positively associated with profits and output which was negatively related to profitability. It is also possible that Labour Governments might have been associated with a negative impact on the profitability of the tobacco industry. For prevention policy, though, the empirical results were particularly interesting for the variables which were not statistically significant. Neither Health Education Council spending nor health warning shocks appeared to have any impact on current profitability. Also changes in real tax yields have not affected the tobacco industry's profit rates. In this model, the statistical tests provided no support for the claims that increased taxation reduces profitability.

A further statistical study was undertaken into the determinants of profitability at the level of individual companies. Here, the interest was on the effects of diversification on profitability. Diversification is of major concern to both companies and policy-makers. It is one method by which firms can protect themselves and adjust to government prevention policies aimed at reducing both smoking and drinking. A single equation statistical model was tested in which company profitability depended on company output, labour productivity and the percentage of shares held by the largest named shareholder. Also, diversification variables were included based on the percentage of business outside the firm's main activity and the proportion of turnover earned outside the UK. In the model, shareholding was used to indicate the extent of separation between ownership and control; the hypothesis being that manager-controlled enterprises will pursue objectives other than maximum profits. Ambiguities surround the diversification variables. Diversification into more profitable industries and overseas markets results in a positive relationship. However, diversification may have no effect or might be more than offset if a company's main product is declining (e.g. tobacco), or if overseas markets are more competitive than the home market.

172

The statistical model was tested using cross-section data for 27 brewers and 4 tobacco companies in 1984 (see Table 8.5). For the combined sample of all companies, diversification was found to have a significant and positive effect on profitability, but the result was sensitive to the inclusion of the tobacco firms. There was also some tentative support for shareholding having the expected positive effect on profitability, although once again the result depended on the inclusion of the tobacco companies in the sample. To further explore the role of diversification, a time-series study was undertaken of two tobacco companies, namely Gallaher and Imperial, using data for 1970-85. For both companies, there was evidence of reduced dependence on tobacco sales favourably affecting profitability. Thus, on the basis of these empirical tests, there was some support for the hypothesis that diversification leads to improved company profitability. It is, of course, likely that diversification by the tobacco companies reflects their response to actual and expected prevention policies and so, indirectly, explains the lack of any relationship between taxation and industry profitability. Diversification also raises wider policy issues about monopoly power and the creation of large enterprises which are potentially powerful producer groups able to influence consumer tastes and government policy in their favour.

POWER, INFLUENCE AND PUBLIC POLICY

What is the policy problem?

The traditional focus of economic analysis of the alcohol and tobacco industries fails to take into account the health implications and wider social aspects of smoking and drinking. Questions arise as to whether the UK alcohol and tobacco industries are socially desirable and whether their outputs are too large or too small. An individualistic and laissez-faire analysis assumes that markets function efficiently without government policies. An alternative view suggests that, if left to themselves, private markets will fail to work properly and that state intervention is required to correct market failures. Markets might fail because of harmful or beneficial external effects (e.g. pollution, street lighting) or because of imperfections in the form of monopolies, oligopolies and entry barriers. These polarised approaches lead to conflicting objectives for alcohol and tobacco policy. Supporters of individual consumer choice and market solutions will favour de-regulation, liberalisation and competitive markets which will lead to lower prices and a larger output compared with monopoly. However, supporters of reduced smoking and drinking might welcome the higher prices and output restrictions associated with monopoly power! There are, then, potential conflicts between competition policy, health and prevention policies. To understand some of the policy issues, it is necessary to know whether the UK alcohol and tobacco industries are monopolistic and whether their behaviour is against the public interest.

Acting against the public interest

Critics of the alcohol and tobacco sectors can find much in the industrial structure and in the conduct of the enterprises to support their case. Both are oligopoly industries dominated by a small number of firms which are large in relation to the size of the market. The major firms in both industries are also large in terms of their absolute size (Table 8.3). With small numbers of firms, collusion is more likely and competition often takes the form of non-price strategies such as brand proliferation, advertising, marketing and sponsorship. These strategies themselves generate barriers to entry. For example, Imperial Tobacco (Hanson Trust) incorporates John Player, Wills and Ogdens and its leading cigarette brands include Superkings, John Player Special, Regal King Size, Embassy, Woodbine and Lambert and Butler. Similarly, Bass, for example, offers a variety of regional brands such as Stones, Bass Special, Worthington, Allbright, Toby and Tennant beers. Brands have to be advertised. For the brewers, the advertising to sales ratio almost doubled from 1.5 per cent in 1960 to nearly 3 per cent in 1983. Whilst for the tobacco companies, the advertising to sales ratio remained around 1 per cent throughout the period (see Chapter 2). Critics claim that large-scale advertising forms a barrier to entry, but an alternative view regards advertising as a means of providing valuable information to consumers. Of course, advertising, especially of cigarettes, has been subject to various restrictive voluntary agreements. Firms are likely to respond to restrictions by searching for alternative methods of marketing such as the employment of more sales staff and the extension of sponsorship.

The brewers are involved in a further aspect of non-price competition through their tied-houses which have been criticised as a restriction on competition and an additional barrier to new entry into the industry (Cowling, 1980). Indeed, the 1969 Monopolies Commission Report on the Supply of Beer concluded that in England and Wales the tied-house system operated against the public interest. The Commission argued that the restrictions on competition involved in the tied-house system operated by the brewers were:

'... detrimental to efficiency in brewing, wholesaling and retailing, to the interests of independent suppliers (including potential new entrants) and to the interests of consumers' (Cmnd. 216, 1969, p.119).

To remedy defects in the tied-house system, the Monopolies Commission recommended that the licensing system in England and Wales should be substantially relaxed. These are interesting conclusions in the context of current debates about liberalisation, de-regulation, the licensing laws and competition in the brewing industry. The Monopolies Commission's conclusions also suggest that the monopoly associated with the tied-house system is policy-created! As always, though, markets find alternative solutions and competition has emerged through the expansion of alternative outlets (e.g. supermarkets, clubs).

Whilst critics of the alcohol and tobacco industries can point to many aspects of conduct which they condemn, they have to work within the framework of current UK monopoly and competition policy. This involves a two-stage approach concerned with identifying a monopoly situation and then determining whether it is acting against the public interest. UK policy defines a monopoly as a situation where 25 per cent of the market is supplied by one firm or by a group of firms acting together or is likely to result from a proposed merger. In addition, mergers can be referred to the Monopolies and Mergers Commission if the assets involved exceed £30 million. On this basis, the high concentration ratios in the tobacco industry suggest a monopoly situation, with Imperial and Gallaher each with over 25 per cent of the UK market (Booth et al., 1986). Moreover, the tobacco industry's profitability has usually exceeded the national average which could indicate monopoly profits (Table 8.7). Against these points, though, it has to be recognised that the UK industry's output has been declining and that there is competition from foreign firms and from Rothmans which increased its share of the UK market from under 6 per cent in 1963 to 15 per cent in 1984. Furthermore, recent developments in economic theory suggest that in assessing industrial efficiency, much greater emphasis should be given to the opportunities for contestibility through actual and potential rivalry rather than focusing on the existing number of firms in an industry (Baumol, 1982).

The UK brewing industry is not as highly concentrated as the tobacco industry. Indeed, none of the leading brewers had 25 per cent or more of the market which is the UK policy definition of a monopoly situation. Nor does there appear to be any evidence of monopoly profits; the industry's profit rates have usually been below the national average. However, the tied-house system remains controversial. Moreover, it has to be recognised that even if a firm has monopoly power, it might choose not to exercise it, because it wishes to deter new entrants or because it is concerned with objectives other than maximum profits. There is also one distinctive feature of both the major brewers and the tobacco companies, namely, their large absolute size. If absolute size is necessary for creating producer groups able to influence

175

government policy in their favour, then the leading brewing and tobacco companies must be amongst the major interest groups in the UK.

Producer groups

Public choice analysis predicts that the policies of democratic governments tend to favour producers rather than consumers. Producers can combine to form an interest group seeking to influence government policy in their favour. They will lobby against tax increases on their products referring to the jobs and export benefits of their industry. They will try to capture any regulatory agencies for the industry and will seek to ensure that regulation benefits producers rather than consumers. Whilst producer groups have a major role in public choice models, few efforts have been made to operationalise the concept.

Critics of the brewing and tobacco companies claim that they are a powerful and influential pressure group. If so, an analysis of the major UK companies and their market environment provides insights into the characteristics of powerful producer groups. The UK brewing and tobacco industries are dominated by a small number of firms and small numbers facilitate agreement on key issues. For example, both industries have made voluntary agreements over advertising restrictions. The major firms are also large both in relative and absolute size and have an international business. Products are highly differentiated and supported by extensive advertising. In the case of tobacco, the industry is highly concentrated and characterised by large conglomerates. The industries have established a degree of vertical integration, either forward into retail or backward into raw materials. Both brewers and cigarette companies have specialised trade associations (Brewers Society and Tobacco Advisory Council), each of which is involved in lobbying, advertising and public relations on behalf of their industry. The structure-performance model examined earlier, implies that some of these characteristics may have emerged as a response to government policy. The current strength of producer groups may therefore be a function of past restrictive policy.

CONCLUSION

Government prevention policy on tobacco aims to reduce the harm associated with smoking through reducing consumption. Public concern is also now focusing on alcohol prevention policy and the likely effects on public health and public order of increased availability. In the past, both policy and analysis have centred on affecting the demand for alcohol and tobacco.

However, the supply side has been shown to be a major factor affecting policy success. Producer groups lobby to minimise the impact of potential restrictive policy and firms act to neutralise the actual effect of current and expected restrictive policy. These feedback effects may constitute a direct impediment to control policy aimed at availability and supply. However, they may also indirectly impede control policy aimed at consumers, as any reaction by firms will affect the market conditions in which consumers make their choices. Demand and supply are interactive forces in the markets for alcohol and tobacco products.

Ultimately, the response of firms to prevention policies depends on the impact on profitability, balanced against the power of producer groups and firms to maintain profitability and influence policy. If the power of producer groups is limited, policies which reduce the profits to be earned in the alcohol and tobacco sectors will result in a shift of investment to other sectors so that output will decline. However, one response to restrictive policy may be to increase producer group power rather than to shift investment. This will continue for as long as potential profits from continued investment exceed the costs of gaining greater lobby influence. Evidence in the brewing and tobacco sector suggests that increased concentration, combined with diversification to reduce risk, may have maintained (if not increased) lobby group power while also helping to maintain profitability in the presence of prevention policy. Although the empirical evidence is limited due to inadequate data sources, the implications are clear. A supply side analysis is an essential component of any comprehensive evaluation of prevention policy.

Notes

1. Some of the material for this chapter (e.g. on ownership) was collected by Roy Boakes, Research Fellow, Addiction Research Centre, University of York. Valuable comments were received from Christine Godfrey, Alan Maynard and David Robinson: the usual disclaimers apply.

2. Multiple regression equations were estimated in both linear and log-linear forms.

References

Baumol, W. et al., (1982), *Contestable Markets and the Theory of Industry Structure*, Harcourt Brace Jovanovich, London.

Booth, M., Hardman, G. and Hartley, K., (1986), 'Data Note 6, The UK alcohol and tobacco industries', *British Journal of Addiction*, 81, 825-830.

Booth, M., Boakes, R., Hartley, K. and Hardman, G, (1988), 'Data Note 14, Mergers in the UK alcohol and tobacco industries', *British Journal of Addiction*, 83, 707-714.

Brewers Society, (1986, 1988), Statistical Handbook , London.

Brouwer M.T., (1981), 'The European beer industry', in de Jong, H. W. (ed.), *The Structure of European Industry*, Martinus Nijhoff, The Hague.

Cockerill A., (1977), 'Economies of scale, industrial structure and efficiency: the brewing industry in nine nations', in Jacquemin, A. and de Jong, H. W. (eds.), *Welfare Aspects of Industrial Markets*, Martinus Nijhoff, The Hague.

Cmnd. 216, (1969), *Report on the Supply of Beer*, Monopolies Commission, April, HMSO, London.

Cmnd. 7198, (1978), *A Review of Monopolies and Mergers Policy*, HMSO, London.

Cooper, R., Hartley, K. and Harvey, C., (1970), *Export Performance and the Pressure of Demand*, Allen and Unwin, London.

Cowling, K. et al., (1980), *Mergers and Economic Performance*, Cambridge University Press, Cambridge.

Cubbin, J. and Leach, D, (1983), 'The effect of shareholding dispersion on the degree of control in British companies: theory and measurement', *Economic Journal*, June.

EAG, (1969), *The Economics of Brewing*, Economists Advisory Group, London,

Kirzner, I., (1973), *Competition and Entrepreneurship*, University of Chicago Press, Chicago.

Meeks, G., (1977), *Disappointing Marriage: A Study of the Gains from Merger*, Cambridge MP, Cambridge.

Pratten, C.F., (1971), *Economies of Scale in Manufacturing Industry*, Cambridge MP, Cambridge.

Rees, R.D., (1973), 'Optimum plant size in UK industries: some survivor estimates', *Economica*, November.

Scherer, F.M., (1973), 'The determinants of industrial plant sizes in six nations', *Review of Economics and Statistics*, LV, 2.

Scherer, F.M., (1980), *Industrial Market Structure and Economic Performance*, Rand McNally, 2nd Edition, London.

Scouller, G., (1987), 'The UK merger boom in perspective', *National Westminster Bank Quarterly Review*, May.

9 Prevention policy and the Scotch whisky industry

MARK BOOTH AND RON WEIR

Those who advocate measures designed to reduce the level of alcohol consumption quite naturally stress the benefits which might follow; benefits such as an improvement in personal health, the reduction in the number of working days lost through alcohol related illnesses, and greater safety on the roads. The attainment of such benefits is not costless, for a reduction in total alcohol consumption implies a reduction in demand for the products of the alcoholic beverage industries, and a consequential loss of employment and remuneration for those who earn a livelihood in the drinks industry, either directly as producers and distributors, or indirectly as suppliers of raw materials and intermediate goods. In other words a potential conflict exists between two objectives, namely improvements in health status (as well as other indicators of social well- being) and wealth creation through the income and employment generated by the drinks industry. Such conflict could remain potential rather than actual if, for example, higher taxes on alcohol reduced per capita consumption but population growth stabilised or expanded total demand, or if a reduction in home demand was offset by an increase in export demand. Policy makers need to be aware of the nature of the trade-off between prevention and wealth creation. Such an awareness can best be developed, and the nature of the trade-off demonstrated, by an industrial case study. Accordingly, this chapter presents a microeconomic evaluation of the effects of, and the likely responses to, prevention policy in the Scotch whisky industry. The chapter proceeds on the assumption that a prevention policy involving an increase in the real level of excise duty designed to lower alcohol consumption has been implemented. The Scotch whisky industry has been selected for study not because whisky attracts a low rate of excise duty, in fact measured in terms of alcohol content Scotch is more heavily taxed than other alcoholic beverages, but rather because certain features of the industry highlight the conflict between health objectives and wealth creation. These features are as follows.

1. The industry is one of Scotland's largest employers with an estimated 16,000 employees; a major foreign currency earner with exports valued at £1,070 million in 1986; and, one of the most important sources of revenue in the Scottish economy. The regional and national effects of prevention policy can therefore be analysed.
2. Since 1978 the industry has experienced a significant reduction in demand and its reaction to this offers a proximate guide to the likely effects of prevention policy.
3. The pattern of ownership within the industry has altered substantially over the past four years and the motives behind this are relevant for the way in which the industry might react to prevention policy.
4. The industry has a long and successful record in lobbying Parliament and Government.

The chapter begins with a brief description of the production process[1]. The structure of the industry, including recent changes in ownership, is considered next. Trends in production, employment and exports are then established. Taxation policy is reviewed and finally, the descriptive material is used to discuss the implications of prevention policy.

THE PRODUCTION PROCESS

Whisky is a distilled spirit made from cereals, water and yeast. Two types of whisky are produced, malt whisky and grain whisky. Malt whisky is made in pot stills from a mash of malted barley and the process is a discontinuous or batch one. Grain whisky is made by a continuous process in the patent or Coffey still from a mixture of malted barley and unmalted grain, normally maize. Grain whisky costs less to make, is produced in much larger quantities and, in terms of flavour, is a much more homogeneous commodity than malt.

Because the pot still carries over much more flavour of the raw materials than the patent still, malt whisky is a more heterogeneous product than grain. Each production area and, to some extent, each distillery has its own individual characteristics. It is customary to divide producers into four main geographical regions: (a) Lowland malt—made south of an imaginary line drawn from Dundee to Greenock; (b) Highland malt—made north of that line; (c) Islay malt—from the Island of Islay; (d) Campbeltown malt—from Campbeltown in the Mull of Kintyre.

After distillation whisky is matured in oak casks for at least three years, the minimum legal requirement, though in practice normally for a good deal longer.

After maturation the majority of malt and grain whisky is blended to produce standard or de-luxe blended whisky, the difference between the two being the length of time the whisky has been allowed to mature and the proportion of malt in the blend. A blended whisky may contain anything up to fifty different types of whisky. A smaller but increasing quantity of whisky is sold as single malts. Only one grain whisky, Cameron Brig, is actually sold as a single grain. The maturation process introduces a long time interval between production and consumption and the cost of financing whisky stocks means that there can be high financial penalties for firms which over- or under-estimate the future course of demand.

Table 9.1

Average retail price of a bottle of whisky 1986/87

Type	Price[a] £	
Highland malt	14.88	(n = 55; sd = £1.37)
Lowland malt	13.12	(n = 6; sd = £0.95)
Islay malt	15.06	(n = 7; sd = £0.87)
Campbeltown malt[b]	14.40	(n = 2; sd = £3.18)
Vatted malt[c]	12.94	(n = 14; sd = £1.48)
Grain whisky[d]	11.10	
Blended whisky[e]	11.44	(n = 91; sd = £2.44)

a. Price includes VAT at 15%
b. Only 2 Campbeltown malts are produced priced at £16.65 and £12.15
c. A vatted malt is a blend only containing malt whiskies
d. Only one brand of grain whisky is included
e. Blended whisky includes both de-luxe and standard blends
        n = number in sample
        sd = standard deviation

Source: ARC database.

181

With differences in the basic production cost (including maturation) and an important element of product differentation which enables some producers of single malts to obtain higher prices than those who make bulk malts for blending, there is a spectrum of prices as the recommended retail prices from one wholesale supplier in 1986/87 shows (Table 9.1). This pricing has important implications for the way a prevention policy which operated through an increase in the level of excise duty (tax) would influence the demand for different types of whisky with a flat rate duty falling more heavily on the lower priced whiskies.

THE STRUCTURE OF THE INDUSTRY

Although the Scotch whisky industry can be regarded as consisting of a number of separate manufacturing processes—distilling, blending, bottling, broking, coopering—the trend throughout the twentieth century has been for firms to embody all these processes.

The present day industry is dominated by Guinness following its controversial but successful bid for the Distillers Company (DCL) in April 1986. Before this DCL held the dominant position. DCL originated in April 1877 as an amalgamation of six Lowland grain or patent still distilling firms. After 1900 a prolonged contraction of demand, which lasted until 1932, persuaded the DCL to adopt a policy of consolidation or rationalisation in which the firm came to control virtually all the grain whisky distilleries in the United Kingdom and a majority of the pot still distilleries. It also extended its interests into the production of blended whisky during the First World War, a move which threatened a group of blending firms known as 'The Big Three': James Buchanan & Co. Ltd., John Dewar & Sons Ltd. and John Walker & Sons Ltd. In 1915 the first two firms formed a holding company, Scotch Whisky Brands Ltd. later renamed Buchanan-Dewar Ltd. in 1919. Continuing decline in the home market, and tariff barriers and anti-drink campaigns in export markets convinced DCL and 'The Big Three' that a merger would be mutually beneficial. Talks which had started in 1909 and continued spasmodically were concluded in 'The Big Amalgamation' of 1925, the second largest amalgamation by value in British manufacturing industry during the inter-war period. The new DCL group accounted for an estimated 60 per cent of Scotch whisky sales in 1925. Total consumption of home produced spirits in 1925 was 19 million proof gallons (m.p.g.) compared to 128 m.p.g. in 1980. The group formed a suitable organisation for continued acquisitions within the Scotch whisky industry, such as those of White Horse Distillers (1927) and Benmore Distilleries Ltd. (1928), and in the gin distilling trade, such as Booths Distilleries Ltd. (1937). Two other aspects of the group's response to the marketing problems of the inter-war depression are worth noting. One was direct investment in overseas production facilities, for example, in Canada (1927), Australia (1929) and the United States (1934). The other was a substantial amount of diversification mainly into the chemical industry via the production of industrial alcohol and its derivatives but also including products such as plasterboard, anti-freeze and synthetic resins. An important motive behind the amalgamation in 1925 had been the desire to reduce the number of brands of blended whisky and thus the cost of sales promotion in a declining market. Little progress was made with this. Blame has often been placed on the Group's loose federal structure but in fact centralised controls were gradually introduced after 1925 and the main justification for retaining brands lay in the contemporary belief that consumers were loyal to particular brands and would react unfavourably if they were extinguished. A much more serious failure was the Group's inability to rationalise the means of distribution, an issue which did relate to the sovereignty of the subsidiary blending firms[2].

Whisky consumption, at home and abroad, did not pass the peak of 42.8 m.p.g. established in 1900 until 1965. Recovery from the mid 1930s was based on the export market and in volume terms the home market still remains smaller than in the last year of Queen Victoria's reign, a remarkably long term consequence of the anti-drink campaign at the beginning of the twentieth century (Weir, 1984a). Since the Second World War the industry's fortunes have been closely tied to exports (Table 9.2).

With its remarkable success in developing new overseas markets the industry experienced a long period of expanding demand, broken only in 1968 and 1978. Rates of growth were impressive (Table 9.3).

Today the industry exports over 80 per cent of its output, a record not passed by any other UK industry.

Although DCL presided over the politics, production and pricing of the Scotch whisky trade during the forty years after 'The Big Amalgamation', its share of the home market and the degree of concentration in the industry began to decline in the 1960s (Table 9.4). The reasons were twofold. First, small producers such as Arthur Bell & Sons Ltd. and William Teacher & Sons Ltd. began to expand production and to achieve significant sales in the home market. Secondly, the large brewing firms started to buy distilleries to produce whisky for sale in their own outlets. Historically this was not a new phenomenon but the entry of firms such as Scottish and Newcastle Breweries Ltd., who acquired Mackinlay-McPherson Ltd. in 1961, was very difficult to counter by DCL as the new entrants were not small companies that could easily be taken over, but very large diversified companies[3]. The threat of a reference to the Monopolies and Mergers Commission also deterred DCL from attempting to counter these new entrants by its traditional strategy of a

Table 9.2
Consumption of home produced spirits
(million litres of pure alcohol)

Year	(A) Home	(B) Export	(C) Total	% Exports
1900	100.4	14.8	115.2	13%
1920	43.3	18.9	62.2	30%
1930	24.9	16.1	41.0	39%
1940	25.2	30.6	55.8	55%
1950	15.8	25.2	41.0	61%
1960	29.6	60.0	89.6	67%
1970	36.6	160.9	197.5	81%
1980	50.1	249.9	300.0	83%
1986	45.4	236.2	281.6	84%

Col. A: UK consumption of home-produced spirits (this definition includes other types of spirit produced within the UK, mainly gin).

Col. B: For 1900, 1920, 1930 and 1940 the series is for home-produced spirits; for subsequent years, Scotch whisky and Northern Irish whiskey only.

Sources: G. B. Wilson, *Alcohol and the Nation* (London, 1940), App. F, Tables 1 & 8, pp.331–4 and 352–3; W Birnie, *Statistics relating to British made Potable Spirit* (Inverness, 1952); Scotch Whisky Association, *Statistical Reports*. Wilson and Birnie's series were measured in proof gallons and have been converted into litres of pure alcohol.

Table 9.3
Rates of growth of Scotch whisky exports

	Volume	Value
1946–1968	11.1	13.5
1968–1978	5.9	14.1

Source: Scotch Whisky Association, *Statistical Reports*.

take-over bid. An even more fundamental reason for DCL's hesitancy was that it regarded the brewers mainly as competitors in the home market, the slower growing and less profitable section of the trade. By 1970 DCL was earning over 90 per cent of its profits from exports. Nevertheless, DCL did respond to the increasingly competitive conditions in the home market in a variety of ways. It appointed a brewing firm, Bass Charrington, as agent in England and Wales for the brand VAT 69 in order to gain access to the brewer's tied houses. It began to rationalise distribution creating a new subsidiary, Buchanan-Booth's Agencies, for the joint marketing of three brands: Black & White, Booth's Gin and Cossack Vodka. It appointed independent companies as agents for its smaller brands. It sought to meet competition in the off-licensed trade from the growth of supermarkets by developing low-priced blends and, as an alternative to the brewers' tie, introduced group loyalty payments—discounts—for customers whose requirements included a fixed minimum (70 per cent) of DCL's brands.[4] These measures were in the long term inadequate to preserve DCL's share of the home market from the inroads made by brewers' own brands and the aggressive marketing of independents such as Bells and Teachers.

Table 9.4

DCL's estimated share of the home whisky market

1960	75%
1967	50%
1984	20%

Sources: For 1960 and 1967, The Monopolies Commission (1969); for 1984 estimates made during Guinness bid for DCL.

The sharpest reduction on DCL's share of the home market owed nothing to competition from the brewers and everything to competition within the European Community when DCL's dual-pricing policy was struck down by the European Commission in December 1977 and the firm withdrew Johnnie Walker Red Label, the market leader, from the home market.[5]

The long export boom, which lasted until 1978, attracted outside investors to the Scotch whisky industry, both for investment in mature stocks and in productive capacity which rose by an estimated 50 per cent during the 1970s.[6] Such external investment merely acknowledged the fact that Scotch whisky was increasingly coming to be regarded as an internationally tradeable commodity, but it gave rise to concern about the amount of foreign ownership, or external control, in the industry. The number of distilleries owned by foreigners rose from 14 per cent in 1960 to 21 per cent in 1980 against a background of an overall increase in the number of plants (Table 9.5). Brewing firms continued to display an interest in the industry. Whitbread, for example, purchased Long John Distilleries in 1975 and Allied Lyons acquired Teachers. The most fiercely contested bid came in 1985 when Guinness purchased Arthur Bell & Son Ltd. for £360 million.

Table 9.5

Foreign ownership of distilleries 1960–1980

Number of distilleries owned by:	1960	1970	1980
Overseas companies	14	17	24
UK companies	83	92	93
	97	109	117

Source: Monopolies and Mergers Commission 1980 (Cmnd.743)

By 1985 DCL was grappling, belatedly in the minds of many financial commentators, with the problem of excess productive capacity as demand for Scotch whisky declined. Its decentralised management structure in which the key decisions about the main brands were made by the blending subsidiaries and its delegation of management reponsibility in the vital export market to agents with long term contracts, inhibited an effective response. So too did a traditional paternalistic regard of the welfare of the small, isolated communities where many of its distilleries and blending plants were located. In December 1985 DCL was the subject of a hostile bid by Argyll, the first time since 1915 that DCL had been threatened by a takeover bid. DCL turned to Guinness as a 'White Knight' and proposed a £2.19 billion merger. Had this merger gone though it would have given the new firm an estimated 36 per cent of the UK market and 41 per cent of the world market for Scotch whisky. In February, 1986 Argyll raised its bid to £2.7 billion; the Guinness bid was referred to the Monopolies and Merger Commission and was subsequently withdrawn. Guinness then announced a new bid of £2.35 billion plus a promise to reduce the combined firm's share of the UK market to 25 per cent by disposing of ten small whisky companies (25 per cent being the legal definition of a monopoly). The brands were purchased by Whyte & MacKay, the whisky subsidiary of Lonrho, and gave it 16 per cent of the UK whisky market. The Department of Trade and

Industry cleared this bid and the two companies merged in April 1986, an acquisition ultimately valued at £2.7 billion.

For the demise of a firm whose critics had initially concentrated on its declining share of the home market what was surprising about the Guinness bid for DCL was the way in which the bid was presented as an opportunity to strengthen Britain's position in the *international* drinks market. The bid was, in the words of Ernest Saunders, the chief executive of Guinness, an opportunity to create, 'a British-owned international consumer brands company able to compete on even terms with the foreign-owned giants' (*Financial Times,* 1986). The current view in the drinks industry is that ownership of brands is the key to success, the sine qua non in a business that is highly competitive internationally. What lies behind this reasoning is a number of important changes in the market facing drinks producers. The first is the slowing down of economic growth in the major industrialised nations. In the expansion of whisky sales during the 1970s a strong correlation existed between increased income, wealth and spirits consumption. With the downturn in economic activity the ensuing weakness of demand has intensified competition. The second is a shift in consumer preference away from brown spirits towards wine and alternative drinks that are perceived as being healthier. This trend has also been encouraged by the skilful marketing of rival products to whisky such as 'mixer' drinks. Finally, there has been a rapid growth in the production of local whiskies, sometimes marketed as 'Scotch-type' whiskies, and in low-strength, cut-price labels. The future of the drink business in the 1990s in thus seen as one of managing a long-term decline in demand and, it is argued, this is easier to manage on a global scale. The structure of the international drinks industry on this reasoning will therefore consist of a small league of large-scale multinational drinks companies, each with a portfolio of leading brands.[7] The key elements in this structure are already in place (Table 9.6).

Essentially these are arguments about the scale of business necessary to compete successfully in internationally traded commodities and they leave the economist's conventional measuring rods of concentration wanting: what implications can be drawn from the share of an international market held by the top three, five or ten firms? Part of the answer may be found in the decisions taken by these major firms in the aftermath of the merger mania of 1986, for one clear outcome has been the concentration on the core (alcohol beverage) business and the disposal of subsidiaries engaged in activities which are not immediately related to the core. Examples can be found in Guinness's realisation of DCL's carbon dioxide and food interests, as well as its own newspaper and health food interests. Entry costs to the international drinks trade are also high, as Argyll, the unsuccessful suitor for Distillers, pointed out when it disposed of its drink interests: 'it may no

Table 9.6

Estimated operating profits of major drinks companies (wines & spirits excluding beer, 1986)

Company	US$mn	£mn
Guinness Beverage Group (UK)	427	277.3
Grand Metropolitan (UK)	362	235.1
Moet-Hennessy (Fr)	249	161.7
Allied-Lyons (UK)	212	137.7
Seagram (Can)	200	129.9
Brown-Forman (USA)	167	108.4
Suntory (Jap)	127	82.5
Pernod-Ricard (Fr)	126	81.8
Whitbread (UK)	49	31.2

Spirit sales by volume

1. Grand Metropolitan/IDV (UK)
2. Seagram (Can)
3. Guinness (UK)
4. Allied Lyons/Hiram Walker (UK)
5. Suntory (Jap)
6. Bacardi (Bah)
7. Pernod-Ricard (Fr)
8. National Distillers (USA)
9. Brown-Forman (USA)
10. Whitbread (UK)

Source: *Sunday Times,* Business News, 1.3.1987.

longer be practicable in a highly concentrated industry for Argyll to establish a major international drinks business at an acceptable cost' (*Financial Times,* 1987). A corollary to this is the exit from the drinks industry of US National Distillers which decided to sell its wine and spirits business and concentrate on petrochemical and energy marketing, and Beechams disposal of its stake in Eurobrands. Such trading realignments have implications for prevention policy if only because in the past, diversification was seen as a way of responding to decline in the drinks market and, more recently, was the strategy adopted by tobacco firms to the decline in smoking. The large-scale firm has, of course, considerable advantages through the resources it can command in responding to decline in its main market but, at the very least, the increasing concentration on core activity by major drinks firms may be predicted to make their reponse to a prevention policy energetic, both in marketing and lobbying.

These recent major changes in the ownership of Scotch whisky companies and brands are reflected in the production end of the trade. It is extremely difficult to obtain data on the specific companies involved in the acquisition of distilleries over a long period of time but the pattern of ownership in 1978 and 1987 was probably fairly close to that outlined in Table 9.7.

Table 9.7

Company ownership of distilleries 1978–1987

Company	Number of distilleries owned	
	1978	1987
DCL	45	–
Guinness/DCL	–	46
Seagrams (Canada)	9	10
Hiram Walker (Canada)	8	8
Highland Distilleries	5	5
Hawker Siddley	–	5
Whitbread	4	5
Invergordon	5	–
Arthur Bell	4	–
Grand Metropolitan	4	4
Lonrho	3	3
Amalgamated Distilled Products	–	3
William Grant	3	3
Other Brewing Companies	4	2
Other Overseas Companies	7	5
Other Companies Owning one or two Distilleries	10	13
	117	112

Source: 1978 as Table 9.1
1987 authors' estimates.

Although it is clear that the pattern of ownership has changed considerably, the implications for control of production are less obvious because distilleries vary widely in scale of output and most companies are unwilling to reveal information on production levels. At best it is necessary to rely on isolated pieces of information, for example, that the post-amalgamation Guinness group controls 35 per cent of the industry's malt distilling capacity, 43 per cent of grain whisky capacity, 25 per cent of Scotch sales in the UK and 42 per cent of the export market for blended whiskies. Productive capacity has always been a particularly flexible concept in the Scotch Whisky industry and, at a time of below capacity working, ownership of particular plants is a poor guide to control over production. An alternative approach is to estimate the share of the market held by each firm's brands (Table 9.8). Only one of these firms is foreign owned and it would therefore appear that foreign owned companies have had a minimal effect on the domestic market. There is no evidence that foreign owned brands have a particularly high share of export markets.

Table 9.8

Estimated UK whisky market shares 1987 (by volume)

1.	Guinness/DCL	25%
2.	Whyte & MacKay	16%
3.	Allied Lyons	14%
4.	Highland Distilleries	10%
5.	Wm. Grant	7%
6.	Whitbread	2%
7.	Seagrams	2%
8.	Grand Metropolitan	2%
9.	Macdonald Martin	1%
	Top 9 firms	79%

Source: Estimated from Trade Press.

PRODUCTION

It is only possible to obtain production totals in quantity terms and not value terms. Levels of Scotch whisky production between 1951 and 1986 are shown in Table 9.9.

Production of Scotch whisky was very low during the Second World War. After the war domestic consumption was deliberately restricted as part of a government policy to try to increase exports to 'hard currency' markets. Distillers were allocated cereals on the understanding that the ratio of exports to home market releases would be kept at three to one. One consequence was a thriving domestic black market in whisky. Rationing of the home market

Table 9.9

Scotch whisky production 1951–1986

(million litres pure alcohol)

Year	Malt	Grain	Total
1951	33.0	42.7	75.7
1961	68.6	120.2	188.8
1970	149.0	222.1	371.1
1971	159.4	228.3	387.7
1972	176.2	258.8	435.0
1973	199.1	272.0	471.1
1974	214.7	261.7	476.4
1975	178.9	215.3	394.2
1976	167.4	194.9	362.3
1977	171.4	222.1	393.6
1978	209.3	250.0	459.3
1979	203.9	255.1	459.0
1980	177.9	238.0	415.9
1981	110.1	157.9	268.0
1982	96.7	151.0	247.7
1983	93.4	145.7	239.1
1984	99.5	153.9	253.4
1985	104.8	155.8	260.6
1986	103.8	161.1	264.9

Source: Scotch Whisky Association.

did not stop until 1959, although formal government restrictions ended in 1953 (Weir, 1974, pp.122–42). Production then started to increase steadily and with rising home and export demand output grew by an average of 7.5 per cent per annum between 1960 and 1974. Production peaked in 1974 and fell by 24 per cent in the following two years. After a partial recovery to 459.5 million litres in 1978 output declined dramatically, at an annual rate of 14 per cent, to reach a new low of 239.1 million litres in 1983. Since 1983 there has been a very modest upturn in production of 3.5 per cent per annum, but output still remains 44 per cent below its peak in 1974. The rapid decline between 1978 and 1983 reflected heavy over-stocking of mature spirit. One result was that firms either closed or moth-balled distilleries. Since 1980 the number of licensed distilleries in the UK has fallen from 129 to 99. With closures and short time working the labour force was reduced and employment levels fell for the first time in the post-war period.

Very little work has been done on optimal production levels in the distilling industry. The Monopolies and Mergers Commission (1980) noted that in the actual malt distilling process the scope for economies of scale is limited. If a firm wishes to increase capacity it will not increase the size of stills, it will merely replicate them. By contrast, scale economies are important in grain distilling, because of the continuous nature of the process, and in bottling plants where large bottling runs are feasible. Scale is also relevant to marketing and the current belief in the industry is that a turnover of at least 10 million cases is required to support a worldwide network of distributors (Wood, 1987).

EMPLOYMENT

The Scotch Whisky industry often claims to be Scotland's largest employer. In fact this position is now held by the computing and electronics industries with some 44,000 employers. Nevertheless, Scotch remains an important source of employment with some 16,000 employees though this is a considerable reduction on the labour force of 25,000 which the industry sustained in the mid 1970s. Concern about the weakness of DCL's management, and the sensitivity of 'the Scottish lobby' to the bid from Guinness, are reflected in the firm's importance as an employer (Table 9.10).

Table 9.10

Number of employees in DCL 1975–1985

(UK employees only)

1975	20,100
1976	19,450
1977	19,156
1978	19,440
1979	19,900
1980	20,240
1981	19,570
1982	18,125
1983	16,850
1984	14,680
1985	13,200

Source: DCL Annual Reports.

Few recent reliable data are available on employment levels within the industry, however the Distilling Sector Working Group (1978) did a detailed breakdown of employment (Table 9.11).

In 1978 the industry employed 25,316 people. Blending and bottling plants were the most important types of employment with 59 per cent of workers being employed in these processes.

Table 9.11

Manpower employed in the Scotch whisky industry (1978)

Method of employment	Malt distilleries	Grain distilleries	Malt and grain distilleries located together	Other[a] operations	Total
Maltings (located at or separate from distilleries)	216	79	205	–	500
Distilleries (inc. warehousing in distilling locations)	3068	2021	–	–	5089
Maturation/ warehousing (located elsewhere than distilleries)	515	451	325	84	1375
Blending and bottling plants	3426	32	9893	1570	14921
By-products plants	192	134	33	–	359
Management, sales and administration	1336	160	1424	152	3072
Totals	8753	2877	11880	1806	25316

a. Includes manpower employed in blending, bottling, broking and other operations not included in manpower employed returns by distillery owning members.

Source: Distilling Sector Working Group (1978).

Employment data on a time series basis is given in Table 9.12. These data are taken from the Census of Production and cover all employment in spirit distilling and compounding, that is, they include employment in vodka and gin production. In 1978 total employment in this sector was 27,100. From Table 9.11 it is known that employment in Scotch whisky was 25,316 or 93 per cent of total employment in spirit distilling and compounding. Adopting the assumption that this proportion remained constant over time, employment figures for the Scotch whisky industry can be estimated. This is done in the final column of Table 9.12 (in reality the percentage is likely to higher in the earlier years and lower in the 1980s).

Table 9.12

Employment in the spirit distilling and compounding sector 1951–1985

Year	Operatives	AT & C	Total	Scotch Whisky
1951	4.4	0.9	5.3	4.9
1954	9.0	3.0	12.0	11.2
1958	11.4	3.2	14.6	13.6
1963	13.1	3.5	16.6	15.4
1968	15.3	4.6	19.9	18.5
1970	17.3	4.9	22.2	20.7
1971	17.5	5.1	22.6	21.2
1972	17.3	5.4	22.7	21.2
1973/74	18.4	5.6	24.0	22.4
1975	19.2	6.1	26.0	24.3
1976	19.2	6.2	25.4	23.7
1977	19.4	6.5	25.9	24.2
1978	20.2	6.9	27.1	25.3
1979	20.2	6.9	27.1	25.3
1980	19.2	7.0	26.2	24.5
1981	17.3	6.7	24.0	22.4
1982	15.6	6.7	22.3	18.2
1983	13.5	6.0	19.5	18.1
1984	12.2	5.5	17.7	16.5
1985	11.3	5.1	16.4	15.2

Source: Census of Production, various years.

A continual rise in consumption was reflected in increasing employment until the contraction of demand in the late 1970s. The reduction of employment appears to have fallen hardest on operatives, whose numbers fell by 33 per cent between 1978 and 1983, whilst the number of administrative, technical and clerical staff fell by only 13 per cent. This has been attributed to increased marketing efforts by whisky firms and the consequent retention or strengthening of sales forces.

EXPORTS

In volume terms exports peaked in 1978 and have declined by 1.8 per cent per annum since then; the nominal, though not the real value of Scotch whisky exports, continued to increase.

Table 9.13

Exports of Scotch whisky and Northern Irish whiskey[a] (1946–1986)

Years	Volume LPA	Value[b] £m	Value[c] £m
1946	15,261,093	10.60	96.4
1950	25,143,756	26.27	196.0
1955	39,860,191	43.67	266.3
1960	60,066,794	65.56	352.5
1965	102,935,642	107.58	484.6
1970	160,914,668	194.06	700.7
1975	234,274,309	366.62	732.9
1976	238,302,745	436.68	732.9
1978	274,072,934	661.22	849.9
1979	262,420,711	707.41	834.2
1980	249,916,996	746.61	746.6
1981	244,239,375	784.75	701.3
1982	251,277,064	871.60	717.4
1983	227,844,492	858.08	657.1
1984	231,286,678	931.38	698.2
1985	227,988,000	1000.80	741.6
1986	237,209,000	1075.10	795.6

a. Refers to one distillery in Northern Ireland

b. Nominal

c. Real – deflated by RPI (1980 = 100)

Source: Scotch Whisky Association.

There are several forms in which Scotch whisky can be exported:

1. it can be bottled in the UK and exported;
2. it can be exported in bulk and bottled in one of the company's factories overseas;
3. it can be exported in bulk and sold to foreign producers who combine it with local spirits and then sell it in competition with Scotch whisky.

This third type of export has caused considerable controversy. Arguments against this form of export are that it decreases sales of genuine Scotch whisky, damages the image of Scotch whisky and facilitates misrepresentation. Arguments in favour are that bulk exports are an important export earner and that 'admixed' blends may lead people to drink genuine Scotch whisky. Thomson (1979) estimates that if exports of bulk malt whisky ceased then employment would decline by 272. However, if bulk exports of blended whisky were to stop, then employment would increase by up to 2,337 people because of extra employment in bottling. Thomson argues that 'Japanese companies provide the main threat to Scotch Whisky sales in the future. Already they are claiming that the largest selling brand of Japanese whisky is the largest selling brand of whisky in the world. Much of the success of this particular brand of Japanese whisky is due to its Scotch Malt which is imported cheaply in bulk and blended with Japanese spirit prior to blending' (Thomson, 1979).

In terms of world sales of whisky, Scotch whisky is the most popular, followed by American whiskey (Table 9.14).

As stated earlier, however, some 'foreign' whiskies may contain Scotch malt whisky.

The major markets for Scotch whisky have remained fairly constant over the last twenty years. For the whole of the period the USA has remained the single most important market although in percentage terms its importance has declined in recent years. The most important export markets are shown in Table 9.15. The fastest growing market has been Japan, mainly because of bulk exports. Italy is one of the most important markets for single malt whisky. In 1987 Scotch whisky was exported to over 190 different markets. Total export earnings from Scotch whisky have increased from £194 million in 1970 to £1,070 million in 1986 in nominal terms.

Table 9.14

Estimated world sales of whiskies, 1976

Type	Sales per annum (million cases)	World market Share (%)
Scotch whiskies	69.0	34.5
American whiskies	52.0	26.0
Canadian whiskies	30.0	15.0
Japanese whiskies	28.0	14.0
Indian whiskies	9.0	4.5
Thai whiskies	2.0	1.0
Irish whiskies	1.6	0.8
Other	8.4	4.2
	200.0	100.0

Source: Distilling Sector Working Group (1978)

Table 9.15

Major export markets for Scotch whisky (1986)

		Volume	% Total	Value	% Total
1	USA	59.5	25.2	245.5	22.9
2	France	25.4	10.8	108.1	10.1
3	Japan	17.3	7.3	64.7	6.0
4	Italy	13.1	5.5	74.5	6.9
5	Spain	11.3	4.8	54.6	5.1
6	Australia	8.5	3.6	22.5	2.1
7	Fed Rep Germany	7.8	3.3	35.3	3.3
8	South Africa	7.7	3.2	30.1	2.8
9	Belg/Lux	5.6	2.4	27.4	2.6
10	Netherlands	4.8	2.0	22.9	2.1
11	Canada	4.7	1.9	23.9	2.2
12	Brazil	4.4	1.9	12.2	1.1
13	Greece	4.2	1.8	19.4	1.8
14	Sweden	3.7	1.6	14.0	1.3
15	Venezuala	3.2	1.3	25.4	2.4
Total worldwide exports		236.2		1,070.1	

Source: The Scotch Whisky Association, Statistical Report, 1986.

TAXATION POLICY

In common with other alcoholic beverages, whisky attracts high levels of duty in both domestic and export markets. At present between 75 per cent and 80 per cent of the retail price of a bottle of whisky is accounted for by tax; this includes VAT of 15 per cent levied on the total retail price including excise duty (Table 9.16). Taxation on whisky has increased steadily throughout the century, although in more recent budgets excise duty has not been increased and the tax burden has declined in real terms.

Table 9.16

Taxation on Scotch whisky (per 75 cl. bottle)

		of which:
Retail price	£7.50,	
Excise duty	£4.73	(63%)
VAT	£0.97	(13%)
Corporation tax	£0.26	(3.5%)
Production costs	£1.05	(14.0%)
Net profit	£0.49	(6.5%)

Source: *Times,* 15.12.1987

The main pressure group in the industry, the Scotch Whisky Association, has consistently campaigned that the level of duty is disproportionately high. On a comparative basis, measured in terms of duty per centilitre of alcohol, Scotch carries the heaviest tax (Table 9.17) and the industry argues for a tax per degree of alcohol 'in line with fiscal neutrality'. The level of taxation in the UK on Scotch whisky represents a higher percentage of the retail price than in any other of the top eleven world Scotch whisky markets. The Distilling Sector Working Group (1978) noted that: 'This high incidence obviously affects the level of sales, and it is noticeable that the industry's most successful marketing overseas occurs in markets where the level of taxation is more moderate by international standards'.

POSSIBLE REACTIONS TO A PREVENTION POLICY

One of the aims of the Addiction Research Centre is to assess the way an industry might react to a prevention policy that reduced demand for that industry's product. Such a reduction in demand hit the Scotch whisky

Table 9.17

Duty charged per centilitre of pure alcohol for five different types of drink

British fortified wine	9.39p
Beer	8.60p
Imported table wine	8.17p
Imported sherry	8.86p
Scotch whisky	15.77p

Source: Scotch Whisky Association, Statistical Report (1986)

industry in the late 1970s. It was not brought about by prevention policies per se but was associated with the slowing down of economic growth in the advanced industrial nations, the imposition or heightening of tariff barriers in export markets, and a loss of market share both with respect to competing spirits and to other types of alcoholic drinks. It has been argued that the latter was associated with an unfavourable consumer reaction on health grounds to brown spirits, a change in consumer tastes independent of any prevention policy. Regardless of the reasons behind the drop in consumption, recent experience serves as a useful proxy for the effects of a prevention policy.

Whisky producers face a particular problem due to the long maturation period. A reduction in consumption means that producers will be overstocked for many years. The first industry reaction to a fall in consumption is likely to be a reduction in the production of whisky to try to minimise overstocking. This is exactly what happened between 1978 and 1983 when production declined by over 48 per cent, and distilleries were either closed down or moth-balled. This caused immediate redundancies in the industry. Employment in spirit distilling and compounding declined from 27,100 in 1978 to 19,500 in 1983. The great majority of redundancies were operatives (6,700) whilst administrative, clerical and technical staff escaped fairly lightly (900) (i.e. 30 per cent of operatives and 13 per cent of administrative, clerical and technical staff have been made redundant since 1978). Such a split of redundancies is to be expected if companies are reducing production but also trying to sell excess stocks.

The reduction in employment (and income) had secondary effects on the Scottish and UK economies. Because of the geographically isolated nature of the distilling industry, distilleries tend to be located in areas of high unemployment and the curtailment of production further depressed local economies. It also meant a reduction in demand for the inputs that are used to produce Scotch whisky: cereals, glass, packaging, energy, transport etc.

One way to assess the spread effects of job losses in one industry on other industries is by means of employment multipliers. Love (1986) has calculated multipliers from the 1979 Scottish input-output tables.[8] These assess the impact of job losses in the whisky industry on the Scottish economy only. Love gives two main figures: (i) he calculates the multiplier effect of an increase in demand for whisky and estimates that a £1 million increase in demand will increase total employment in all Scottish industries by 65 jobs; (ii) he looks at the multiplier for each new whisky related job and finds a value of 3.0, that is, for every new job created in the industry three more jobs will be created in other industries.

Multipliers work in both ways. Love's analysis implies that the 7,600 job losses in the whisky industry between 1978 and 1983 will have given rise to 22,800 job losses in related industries, giving a total of 30,400 job losses due to the decline in consumption. This analysis is, however, fairly pessimistic and assumes that resources, including labour, remain permanently unemployed. The estimate also includes workers in vodka and gin distilleries. Nevertheless, Love estimates that 7–8,000 jobs have been lost in the Scotch whisky industry alone in recent years. A successful prevention policy implies an increase in redundancies and, at least in the short term, sizeable adjustment problems for supplying industries. How well supplying industries cope is largely determined by the availability of alternative sources of demand for the products they formerly sold to the Scotch whisky industry. For cereal growers, where a high degree of regional specialisation exists and where distillers pay premium prices for good quality malting barley, alternative sources of demand are few and less profitable (Weir, 1974, 1984b). The distilling industry's relationship with agriculture also illustrates another point about the burden of adjustment which is that some of the costs fall outside Scotland, for example, on American and European maize producers. Love's use of the Scottish input-output tables for 1979 provides a means of identifying those industries at greatest exposure to a prevention policy (Table 9.18).

Love's research shows that in the rest of the United Kingdom the greatest burden of adjustment would fall on the glass, brewing and packaging industries (Love, 1986, p.7). Also, because of the large number of transactions within the distilling industry (in mature stocks and new whisky), and between the brewing and distilling industries, a prevention policy would exercise severely depressing effects throughout the drinks sector.

A successful prevention policy may also have the effect of decreasing tax revenue. Table 9.19 shows the tax revenue from spirit expenditure taxes.

It can be seen that in real terms tax revenue has decreased considerably from a peak of £1496 million in 1979 to £1312 million in 1986. A successful prevention policy is therefore not a policy without costs as measured in terms

Table 9.18

Major purchases by the Scotch whisky industry, 1979
(as a percentage of each industry's total domestic output and £mn)

Within Scotland	%	£mn
1 Packaging	26.0	41.6
2 Glass	23.0	16.8
3 Brewing	17.9	39.2
4 Spirits & Whisky	12.0	125.2
5 Agriculture	5.4	61.7
6 Electricity	1.2	8.2
7 Insurance, banking and finance	1.0	2.5
8 Timber	1.0	2.4

Source: Love (1986), Table 1, p.7.

Table 9.19
Tax revenues from spirit expenditure

Year	Revenue £mn	Real revenue[a] (1980 prices) £mn
1975	709	1358
1976	902	1493
1977	890	1282
1978	1065	1405
1979	1288	1496
1980	1388	1388
1981	1483	1331
1982	1565	1293
1983	1663	1308
1984	1733	1301
1985	1885	1345
1986	1905	1312

a. Revenue deflated by "all items" Index.

Source: National Income and Expenditure, CSO

of employment and impact on supplying industries. Given, however, that the home market for Scotch whisky is a small proportion of total demand perhaps the key issue is whether measures designed to reduce spirit consumption in the UK would have a harmful effect on exports. If total demand were growing and the industry operating at full capacity it could be argued that a restriction of home demand would merely free output for the export trade, but clearly this is not the present condition of the Scotch whisky industry. Three different possible effects on exports can be identified:

1. 'the shop window effect': this argues that the home market, although small, is an important 'shop window' or advertisement for the industry's products. Brands which are unsuccessful at home are unlikely to do well in export markets; brands which became unavailable because of curtailment of home spirit consumption would stand no chance of being exported.
2. 'the imitation argument': this argues that Scotch whisky faces severe competition in export markets from other spirits, many of which are locally produced. A policy of curbing spirits consumption in Britain, particularly if it were carried out through steep increases in excise duty, would provide a marvellous excuse for governments in countries which import Scotch to protect their own industries by increasing taxation on imported Scotch.
3. 'the scale economies argument': here the proposition is that the home market contributes to reducing the overall production and marketing costs of Scotch whisky and, by doing so, helps Scotch to retain a competitive edge in export markets. A reduction in the home market because of a prevention policy would, therefore, directly damage exports.

Finding suitable evidence and formulating hypotheses to test these propositions are both extremely difficult but the recent structural changes in the industry with their emphasis on the need to create large scale firms with a portfolio of brands together with the rationalisation of production suggest that the scale economies argument is a valid one. The question for advocates of a prevention policy must therefore be whether the benefits from restricting consumption at home are worth the direct costs identified by input-output studies and the risk of damage to the industry's export trade.

Notes

1. For a fuller description of the production process see the Distillers Company Ltd (1966), pp.22–39 and Daiches, D. (1969), pp.1–28.
2. The above discussion is based on DCL's archives and unpublished work by one of the authors.

3.	For the history of relations between brewers and distillers see Weir, R. B. (1974), pp.35–7. For developments in the 1960s see the Monopolies Commission, Beer, (1969), paras. 61–74.

4.	Discussion of DCL's response to competition in the home market based on DCL, Annual Reports and the Monopolies Commission, Beer, page 151.

5.	Dual pricing: DCL's sales strategy in Europe was to appoint a sole distributor for each brand, encourage the distributor to spend on sales promotion, and allow the distributor to sell at relatively high prices. The system only worked if the distributor could not be undercut by any other distributor selling DCL's brands. Supplies to British firms which wished to sell in Europe were therefore either restricted or invoiced at the higher European price.

6.	See Weir, (1974), pp.146–8; and Love, J. H. (1986), page 2. Expansion of capacity during the 1960s may have been even more rapid.

7.	See, Ivan Fallon, 'Genius', *Sunday Times* 1.6.1986; Claire Dobie, 'Strong Scotch may be needed for Distillers', *Independent* 21.1.1987; Liza Wood, 'Everybody is after the same Cocktail', *Financial Times* 4.7.1987.

8.	Employment multipliers: an increase/decrease in the output of industry A will require it to increase/decrease purchases from other industries. These industries in turn will increase/decrease their purchases from other industries. Hence, there is a multiplier effect. The multiplier measures the impact of a change in final demand in industry A on output and employment in the whole economy. See Love (1986), page 10.

References

Daiches, D., (1969), *Scotch Whisky*, Andre Deutch, London.
Distillers Company Limited, (1966), *DCL and Scotch Whisky*, Distillers Company Limited, London.
Distillers Sector Working Group, (1978), *Distilling: Scotch Whisky,* HMSO, London.
Financial Times, (1986), 19th April.
Financial Times, (1987), 17th February.
Love, J.H., (1986), *The Whisky Industry in the Scottish Economy*, Fraser of Allander Institute, University of Strathclyde.
Monopolies and Mergers Commission, (1969), *Beer, A Report on the Supply of Beer*, Cmnd. 216, London, HMSO.
Monopolies and Mergers Commission, (1980), *Hiram Walker Gooderham and Worts Ltd. and the Highland Distilleries Co. Ltd.,* Cmnd. 743, London, HMSO.
Thomson, J.K., (1979), *Should Scotland Export Bulk Whisky?*, Scottish Council for Development and Industry, Edinburgh.
Weir, R.B., (1974), *The History of the Malt Distillers Association of Scotland*, Elgin, London.
Weir, R.B., (1984a), 'Obsessed with moderation: the drinks traders and the drink question (1870–1930)', *British Journal of Addiction*, 79, 93–107.
Weir, R.B., (1984b), 'Distilling and Agriculture (1870–1930)', *Agricultural History Review*, 32, 49–62.
Wood, L., (1987), *Financial Times,* 4th July.

10 Employment

CHRISTINE GODFREY AND KEITH HARTLEY

Prevention policies will be opposed by those groups likely to lose from any change. Consumers and producers are obvious groups likely to suffer from effective prevention policies. Amongst producers, potential losers include shareholders, managers and workers in the UK and overseas. Critics of prevention policies will stress their adverse effects on employment both directly in the industries affected and elsewhere in the economy. References will be made to job losses, their impact on local economies and to the wider employment effects associated with reduced business in supplying industries, in advertising agencies and in the transport and distribution sectors (e.g. shops, public houses). Clearly, opponents of prevention policies whose future income depends on the continued sales of alcohol and tobacco have every incentive to exaggerate the likely job losses. This is an issue dominated by myths and emotion. Informed public choices on prevention policies require careful and independent analysis, critical evaluation and an appraisal of the evidence.

This chapter presents a framework for evaluating the various employment aspects of prevention policies.[1] It outlines the economic determinants of employment and the relationship with unemployment; and it presents and evaluates the available evidence on employment in the alcohol and tobacco industries. There is also an assessment of the arguments and evidence about the total number of jobs both directly and indirectly associated with alcohol and tobacco. Throughout, the aim is to specify the policy-relevant questions, consider the available evidence and identify the gaps in our knowledge.

FRAMEWORK FOR EVALUATION

An information system

In formulating prevention measures, policy-makers need a framework for evaluating their likely effects. They need to know the number of jobs likely to be lost, the type of job (e.g. skill, full- or part-time), their location, and the likely effects on local unemployment rates. Table 10.1 sets out an information system for assessing the employment effects of alternative prevention policies. The table is illustrative rather than comprehensive. It shows three possible policy measures which can be applied to alcohol and/or tobacco products. Additional policies can be included with a more detailed specification of each policy (e.g. tax increase of, say, 10 per cent on the product). Each policy will have a different immediate impact on various sectors of the industry. For example, higher taxes on cigarettes might be shifted to consumers in higher prices, or shifted to workers in the tobacco industry or to shareholders, or even to overseas suppliers. In contrast, a ban on cigarette advertising will have an immediate impact on the advertising agencies, on their outlets (e.g. newspapers) and ultimately, on consumption and hence on the tobacco industry. Similarly, more restrictive licensing laws on the number of premises and their opening times will immediately affect the retailing sector (see Chapter 2).

The approach in Table 10.1 is, of course, a counsel of perfection, which ignores at least two major features of the real world. First, reliable data might not be available for a fully-informed choice. Secondly, policy decisions are made in the political market place with governments seeking votes for re-election, bureaucracies aiming to protect or increase their budgets, and producer groups concerned with their income prospects. Where governments are vote-conscious, then producer groups have every incentive to attribute all job losses to prevention policies. Groups such as management, trade unions and professional and trade associations, concerned about their jobs and income prospects are likely to be a major impediment to vote-sensitive governments seeking to introduce more effective prevention policies (see Chapters 6 and 7). Myth and reality need to be separated. Economists can contribute to the debate through their models of employment and unemployment.

Table 10.1

An information framework

Policies	Direct	In-direct (by indus-try)	Number of Job Losses						
			Total numbers	By skill (managers, skilled unskilled)	By sex (male, female)	Full- or part-time	Location in UK (by region or town)	Local unem-ploy-ment rate (%)	Average wage of those losing jobs (£)
1 Increased taxation									
2 Advertising restrictions									
3 Other regulatory policies (eg, licensing laws)									

Why job losses?

In considering the job effects of prevention policies, it has to be recognised that employment depends upon a variety of factors. To economists, a firm's level of employment is determined by its output, the amount of capital used (e.g. factory, machinery), the level of technology, wage rates and the price of capital. In this model, firms in an industry will reduce employment in response to a fall in output, or an increase in wage rates (labour becomes more expensive), or if machinery becomes cheaper, or if new technology is labour-saving (e.g. computers and word-processors). The model can be modified to allow for firms laying off unskilled labour but retaining skilled labour whose training costs have been borne by the company. Similarly, trade unions can have a role in employment determination through their effects on the level of wages and through restrictive practices designed to protect their members from the job-displacing effects of new technology and new equipment. On this basis, considerable caution is required in assuming a causal relationship between a new prevention policy, such as higher taxation, and job losses. Various other factors can explain job losses. Thus a firm seeking to make the maximum possible impact on a vote-sensitive government has every incentive to attribute all job losses to, say, higher taxation. In these circumstances it is necessary to ask what would have happened to employment in the absence of the new prevention policy?

Some limited tests were undertaken of the basic economic model of employment determination. Initially, a simple model was estimated in which employment was determined by output and technology.[2] The results were statistically significant but based on a limited data set and a restricted model. For the UK brewing industry the model suggested that technical change might have resulted in the loss of 2,500–3,000 jobs per annum for the period 1963–83. Similarly, for the UK tobacco industry during the same period, the estimates showed that technical change resulted in some 600 job losses per annum. The empirical results from these limited tests can also be used to estimate the employment effects of a lower output (see Table 10.1). For a 20 per cent reduction in output, it was estimated that employment might fall by between 4,700 and 7,400 in the UK brewing industry and by some 2,300–4,500 in the tobacco industry.

The simple estimating model was modified and re-estimated in a more complex version.[3] For brewing, the results indicated sluggish short-run employment behaviour with a 1 per cent reduction in total output leading to a 0.4 per cent fall in employment in the first quarter. However, in the long-run, a 1 per cent fall in output is associated with a 1 per cent reduction in employment. The results also confirmed that technical progress has led to job losses in brewing. The more complex model failed to provide a satisfactory explanation of variations in employment in the UK tobacco industry.

When assessing the employment effects of prevention policies, economists will use their models to follow through the relationship between a policy change and its eventual impact on jobs and, ultimately, on unemployment. To industrialists, workers and trade unions in the alcohol and tobacco industries, it is often claimed that more effective prevention policies mean reduced consumption of these products, which in turn is supposed to result in job losses and hence increased unemployment. This model which is summarised in Figure 10.1, leaves much to be desired.

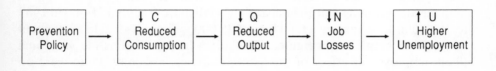

Figure 10.1: Prevention policies and unemployment

The model in Figure 10.1 assumes a set of relationships which link prevention policy to unemployment. However, each link in the chain might be suspect. At the outset, a new prevention policy measure might not be effective in reducing consumption. For example, industry might lobby successfully to modify the penal aspect of a new policy, or it might capture any new regulatory agency, or it can respond with increased advertising. Even if the new policy reduced UK consumption of the product, it does not follow that the output of UK producers will fall (see Chapters 1 and 8). The new policy might reduce imports so that the employment effects will occur outside the UK. Or, if UK consumption falls, domestic producers might respond by increasing exports of their existing products or by diversifying into new product markets (e.g. tobacco companies: see Chapter 8). Even if there is a fall in the output of UK firms, the resulting job losses could be offset by workers accepting lower wages. Finally, whether job losses result in higher unemployment depends upon a variety of factors such as alternative employment prospects and how well and quickly local labour markets are working (for example, via labour mobility or adjustments in wages).

This analytical structure can now be used to interpret some of the facts about employment in the UK alcohol and tobacco industries. Policy-makers need to know how many jobs are likely to be lost from various prevention measures and whether the job losses are likely to be concentrated on, say, unskilled, part-time, non-unionised workers located in areas of high unemployment and possibly in marginal constituencies. The actual effects of prevention policies are estimated from over 20 year's experience of various attempts at health warnings, advertising controls and tax increases, although it is recognised that these series of measures do not necessarily constitute a co-ordinated and effective prevention policy (see Chapter 4).

EVIDENCE

How many jobs are involved?

The total numbers and trends in employment in the UK alcohol and tobacco industries are shown in Table 10.2. Throughout the period, employment in both the alcohol and tobacco industries has fallen from some 151,000 in 1963 to 76,000 in 1986, giving a total loss of 75,000 jobs equivalent to 50 per cent of the 1963 employment figure. This might be regarded as the *maximum* likely employment effect of prevention policies, assuming there were no other influences causing job losses. In tobacco, where for more than 20 years there have been health warnings, education campaigns and fiscal measures all apparently concerned with prevention, industry job losses totalled almost

23,000. However, job losses have been a general feature of the UK economy between 1963 and 1986 and they have not been unique to the alcohol and tobacco industries.

Table 10.2

UK employment

Year	All Manufacturing	Tobacco	Brewing and Malting	Spirits Distilling and Compounding	British Wines Cider and Perry
	(000s)	(000s)	(000s)	(000s)	(000s)
1963	7952	43.3	86.8	16.8	4.2
1968	7826	40.8	80.4	19.9	4.4
1970	8033	39.7	74.5	22.2	5.2
1971	7830	40.7	78.0	22.6	5.5
1972	7522	39.5	70.3	22.7	4.7
1973	7616	39.4	71.6	24.1	4.9
1974	7755	40.2	68.0	26.5	5.1
1975	7467	39.8	66.2	26.0	5.1
1976	7305	37.9	62.0	25.4	5.1
1977	7281	37.7	61.8	25.9	5.2
1978	7106	37.5	61.3	27.1	5.1
1979[a]	6910	37.3	55.9	27.2	5.2
1980	6495	35.7	53.5	26.2	5.0
1981	5778	33.3	47.9	24.0	4.7
1982	5361	31.1	42.8	21.9	4.6
1983	5079	29.8	39.8	19.5	4.3
1984	5059	26.7	37.6	17.7	4.6
1985	4976	23.9	35.6	16.4	4.3
1986	n.a.	20.5	35.3	16.1	4.1

a.   1980 SIC used from this year with new definition of all manufacturing.

Source: *Census of Production,* Business Statistics Office, HMSO (annually).

UK manufacturing industry can be used as an indicator of general trends against which the experience of the alcohol and tobacco sectors can be assessed.   Table 10.2 shows clearly the general downward trend in manufacturing employment, with lob losses throughout the period equivalent to some 37 per cent of 1963 employment levels. On this basis, if alcohol and tobacco had simply followed national employment trends in manufacturing, they might have expected some 56,500 job losses between 1963 and 1985. Allowing for these general downward trends suggests that over the whole period 1963–85, a total of 14,400 job losses in alcohol and tobacco as the maximum likely employment effect of prevention policies (i.e. 70,900 to 56,500). After allowing for national trends, a similar exercise for the tobacco industry over the period 1963–85 indicated some 3,200 job losses as the maximum effect of prevention policies.

Clearly these estimates are extremely crude and simplistic. Much more careful analysis of employment determination in the alcohol and tobacco industries is required. Consideration needs to be given to the employment effects of technical progress in each industry, their extensive involvement in mergers and changing competitiveness in home and overseas markets. Also, as Table 10.2 shows, employment experience has differed within the alcohol industry. Brewing and malting experienced substantial job losses, especially in 1971–72 and between 1978 and 1983; whilst for spirits and wines, 1986 employment levels were similar to those in 1963.

The evidence from industrial employment shows that alcohol and tobacco account for a relatively small proportion of total UK employment in manufacturing, representing 1.9 per cent in 1963 and 1.6 per cent in 1985. In addition, over a considerable period, the maximum total of jobs lost from *all causes* in these industries was some 75,000 or an average of some 3,000 jobs per annum. Such small numbers raise doubts about the reliability of the claims of both industries concerning the likely employment effects of prevention policies, particularly tax increases (see Chapters 3 and 5). However, the industries respond by claiming that the true numbers affected are considerably greater than direct employment in the alcohol and tobacco industries. Moreover, even if the absolute numbers are small in relation to total UK employment, they might well be significant for particular localities.

How many other jobs depend on alcohol and tobacco?

Total numbers employed *directly* in the UK alcohol and tobacco industries were under 80,000 in 1986. There are, though, a number of other jobs which are associated with or indirectly dependent on alcohol and tobacco production. There are jobs in the supplying industries and sectors which form backward linkages. Examples of backward linkages include the growth of cereals (agriculture) for alcohol and the manufacture of specialist machinery and packaging materials for cigarette production. Also, there is employment in the activities which ensure that the manufactured product is delivered to the final consumer, these forming forward linkages. Examples are distribution and retailing. These two sectors have the largest number of jobs claimed to be indirectly linked to alcohol and tobacco.

A study sponsored by the tobacco industry estimated that in 1980 there were 115,000 jobs dependent on the retailing of tobacco (Mackay and

Edwards, 1982). Indeed, the Tobacco Advisory Council has claimed that for every job in the tobacco manufacturing industry, there are seven others dependent on it, mainly in distribution and retailing. The Council has also claimed that between 1980 and 1985 punitive taxation directly contributed to the loss of 50,000 jobs in the tobacco and related industries. Many of these job losses were in areas of high unemployment and have also resulted in the closure of more than 2,000 small retail tobacco businesses (Tobacco Advisory Council, 1985). Not surprisingly, the industry's trade association and the various tobacco retailing associations will seek to persuade governments not to increase taxes on tobacco products (see Chapter 5).

Two methods have been used in previous estimates of the number of indirect jobs dependent on alcohol and tobacco. The first method attempts to identify directly the jobs involved. For example, estimates of the numbers employed in the alcohol industry have included employment in public houses, clubs and restaurants. The second method uses the value of inputs into the industry and outputs, in the form of services rendered, to calculate dependent jobs (MacKay and Edwards, 1982). Estimates based upon both approaches have claimed a far larger number of jobs indirectly dependent on alcohol and tobacco than those directly employed in the industry. However, difficulties arise in estimating indirect employment. There are dangers of double counting, the need to convert part-time jobs to full-time equivalents and the need to obtain reliable estimates of the extent to which jobs actually depend on alcohol and tobacco sales. After examining the advantages and disadvantages of the two methods of calculating indirect employment, consideration is given to changes in indirect employment that may result from government prevention policy.

The direct method of estimating backward and forward employment linkages depends on being able to identify the number employed in processes linked to, but not within, the alcohol and tobacco industries. Certain inputs into these industries may be specialised, such as the manufacture of cigarette machinery or the growth of hops, and this specialisation helps to identify numbers involved. Retail distribution has also been at times a specialised process and the numbers employed in specialist tobacconists and off-licences, for example, could be used. Some of the purchases of the alcohol and tobacco industry are, however, of more general goods such as energy. The usefulness of the direct method therefore depends critically on three factors. First, are estimates of employment available for activities specifically linked to alcohol and tobacco? Secondly, how far are the jobs identified in this way solely dependent on either alcohol or tobacco? Thirdly, how significant a part of the total forward and backward linkages are these identified activities?

211

Several figures are available for employment in retailing alcohol and tobacco. Table 10.3 shows employment in public houses, night clubs, hotels, restaurants and tobacconists. The most noticeable features of this table are the large numbers involved in distribution of these goods. For example, in 1985 employment in public houses was four times larger than the number involved in the production of alcohol. Most of these are part-time jobs (over 75 per cent). Adjusting for part-timers and assuming that two part-time jobs are equivalent to one full-time job, then the 1985 figure of 258,300 actual jobs in public houses is equivalent to 158,700 full-time jobs with a corresponding figure of 161,700 full-time jobs in 1986. As hourly earnings in the service sector are on average considerably lower than manufacturing wages, some care has to be taken in comparisons of the relative size and consequences of changes in employment in the manufacturing and service sectors. It must also be remembered that jobs in night clubs, restaurants and hotels are often associated with activities other than alcohol consumption. Even public houses offer a range of other products and services, especially food.

Table 10.3
Employment in retailing[b]

Year	Public Houses (000s)	Night Clubs etc. (000s)	Hotels (000s)	Restaurants (000s)	Confectioners and Tobacconists (000s)
1971	174.2	81.9	218.7	150.6	n.a.
1975	229.8	99.0	255.0	162.8	n.a.
1979	259.7	113.9	277.8	179.3	n.a.
1980	267.9	117.3	271.2	184.4	n.a.
1981	247.4	116.3	256.7	174.1	n.a.
1982[a]	233.6	141.7	235.0	187.4	155.3
1983	231.0	140.1	234.4	182.7	154.9
1984	241.9	148.4	251.9	189.2	157.8
1985	258.3	155.8	263.2	192.8	160.2
1986	263.2	156.2	273.9	196.2	164.0

a.   Introduction of 1980 SIC.
b.   Figures are for GB only.

Source: Department of Employment, *Employment Gazette,* HMSO, London (monthly).

There are, of course, other jobs involved in the distribution and retailing of alcohol and tobacco. For alcohol, it is necessary to allow for employment in off-licensed premises (36,000 persons in 1984), as well as jobs in supermarkets and mixed retail stores. Tobacco is also sold in supermarkets, food stores, newsagents and off-licences. These examples illustrate the difficulties of estimating indirect employment, particularly in non-specialist businesses. For example, how much of a newsagent's employment should be attributed to tobacco sales? Nor can backward employment linkages be ignored.

The alternative method of estimating indirect employment relies on identifying the flows of backward and forward linkages using the official input-output tables. These trace the inter-relationships between different industries. They show the purchases of the alcohol and tobacco industries from all other industries in the UK and overseas, including the subsequent purchases of these other industries and so on throughout the economy. It is like throwing a stone into a lake and measuring all the ripple effects as these spread throughout the lake. This process of tracing inputs is presented in Table 10.4 which shows that in 1984 the alcohol industry used relatively more inputs from other UK industries than the tobacco industry per unit of output.

The figures of Table 10.4 lead to maximum estimates of indirect employment of 117,400 and 20,700 full-time equivalent jobs (FTEs) for alcohol and tobacco respectively. These estimates are much lower than those claimed by industry, some of the difference reflecting problems in estimating employment in the retailing sector (Godfrey and Hardman, 1987). However, various estimates can be obtained using alternative assumptions (Godfrey and Hartley, 1988). These estimates of total employment, i.e. direct plus indirect employment, range from 345,100 to 429,300 FTEs for alcohol and 79,200 to 162,900 FTEs for tobacco. The corresponding ranges for multipliers (i.e. the ratio of total employment to direct employment) are 5.9 to 7.3 for alcohol and 3.0 to 6.2 for tobacco. Similar calculations for 1968, 1974 and 1979 suggest that these multipliers have changed over time with the multipliers for alcohol rising during the period (Godfrey and Hartley, 1988). These variations suggest that there are dangers in applying constant employment multipliers to predict the effects of prevention policy.

The UK brewing industry has claimed an employment multiplier of 8.5 (Brewers Society, 1985) whilst the tobacco industry has suggested a multiplier of 7.5. For the EC tobacco industry in 1982 there were some 15 jobs (direct and indirect) for every person employed directly in the tobacco industries. However, when these figures are converted to full-time equivalents (FTEs), the employment multiplier for the EC tobacco industries was about six and for the UK, the multiplier was almost five for FTEs

213

Table 10.4

Total requirements per 1,000 units of final industrial output in terms of gross output

Industry SIC Group	Alcoholic Drink	Tobacco
0. Agriculture, forestry and fishing	175.8	35.9
1. Energy and water supplies	102.8	37.1
2. Other mineral and ore extraction. metal manufacturing, chemicals, etc.	108.8	23.2
3. Metal goods, engineering and vehicles	108.8	40.2
4. Other manufacturing		
Total	1333.8	1173.4
Alcohol	1176.1	0.1
Tobacco	0.1	1000.1
5. Construction	24.7	6.9
6. Distribution, hotels, catering, repairs	60.0	30.5
7. Transport and communications	95.3	59.5
8. Banking, finance and insurance	230.7	214.4
9. Other services	14.8	8.7
TOTAL	2255.2	1630.2
Import requirement[a]	58.1	220.2

a. Imports are given in terms of commodity use, not total requirements for each £1000m of output.

Source: Central Statistical Office, 1984, *Input Output Tables for the United Kingdom,* HMSO, London.

(Mackay, 1985, pp.7–8). These employment multipliers are much higher than those for other UK industries where multipliers in the range of two to four have been estimated. A simple check on the claims of the brewing and tobacco industries can be made by considering the ratio of total employment in the UK to employment in manufacturing. In 1984, there were almost four jobs in the economy for every one in manufacturing. Such a wide variety of estimates suggests the need for considerable caution in accepting some of the higher employment figures proposed by the brewing and tobacco industries. Clearly, these groups have every incentive to over-estimate the importance of their industries for employment in the UK. For our purposes, it is accepted that both the alcohol and tobacco industries create indirect jobs and that there are genuine difficulties in obtaining reliable estimates of the numbers involved.

Critics of prevention policies suggest that reductions in the output of the UK alcohol and tobacco industries will not be confined to their industries but will have much wider employment effects throughout the economy. In fact, for the same absolute fall in production, the potential job losses throughout the economy are likely to be greater for reductions in alcohol outputs compared with tobacco, simply because alcohol has a much larger input from other UK industries (Table 10.4). Alcohol employment effects will depend upon how quickly supplying industries are able to readjust and adapt through, for example, entering new markets either at home or abroad. Such adjustments to change are not unique to alcohol and tobacco and have occurred throughout history. Recent examples include the rise and decline of the UK textile, motor-cycle and shipbuilding industries and the emergence of the information technology sector, with the UK economy and the labour market adjusting quite successfully to such changes. When faced with adversity, firms and local communities can be remarkably resilient and prophets of doom and gloom have often been wrong.

The links between levels of consumption and the level of employment in the retailing and distribution sector are much clearer. Often, it is assumed that if the demand for alcohol or tobacco products fell, and no other consumption changed, jobs would be lost. This assumption is, however, difficult to sustain especially in the light of likely prevention strategies. If consumers are persuaded to change consumption habits, by health education, for example, total consumers' expenditure would not fall but would be redistributed between other goods. For retailing, the employment consequences of such changes in taste depend on the comparative labour intensity of selling these substitute goods rather than alcohol or tobacco. If, for example, instead of buying cigarettes from a supermarket consumers switch to wholemeal bread or fresh fruit, more jobs may be needed within the supermarket in packing shelves for each £1 spent on these products rather than cigarettes. Unfortunately, little work has been undertaken on the relative labour requirements of selling different goods or on the goods that may be purchased instead of alcohol or tobacco. It is clear, however, that any large change in tastes could result in costs associated with transition and adjustment. It is not known, for example, how many small shops may depend for their viability on the sale of cigarettes, or how a large shift away from drinking alcohol would affect the public house as a leisure centre. On the other hand, any job losses in the retailing sector are likely to be dispersed over the economy and there will not be the localised effects associated with a factory closure.

215

It is important to note that if the pattern of consumption changes then this may create a new demand for *UK* produced goods. If this is the case then the assumption that no other production rises when tobacco output falls will be invalidated. If consumers buy goods with a large UK content rather than alcohol or tobacco, then new or rather different jobs may be created. Therefore, the overall effect on domestic employment will depend on the changing demand for UK manufacturers and their suppliers and the labour requirements associated with the different consumption patterns.

Calculations of jobs associated with any industry have only a limited usefulness. Indeed, with sufficient ingenuity, it would be possible to carry out a number of studies on the importance of particular industries in employment terms and produce an employment total from these studies that equalled or exceeded the total number employed in the economy! Questions also arise about the type of jobs likely to be lost as a result of effective prevention policies. Are they likely to be skilled or unskilled, men or women, full- or part-time, and are the jobs lost mostly amongst, say, the low paid? Unfortunately, detailed data on these issues are only available for those employed directly in the alcohol and tobacco industries (as shown in Table 10.2).

Are job losses amongst the skilled or unskilled?

If government prevention policies have employment effects, it is important to have some information on the type of jobs that may be lost. For example, some jobs have skills which are transferable and such skills may have a scarcity value even in periods of high unemployment. Other jobs may involve specialised skills which are non-transferable with no alternative use value. Such job losses may require state-supported retraining courses.

Measuring skill levels without detailed knowledge of industrial processes is difficult. Various indicators exist such as the number and ratio of technical to unskilled workers, as well as wage levels. Table 10.5 shows the numbers of operatives, administrative, technical and clerical workers. Care is needed in interpreting these figures since the terms 'operatives', 'technical' and 'clerical' can involve a wide variety of skills. As a rule of thumb, it will be assumed that operatives are relatively unskilled.

Table 10.5 shows that since 1963, most of the job losses in tobacco and brewing, as in manufacturing, have been amongst operatives. Brewing also showed substantial job losses in the administrative, technical and clerical groups. In contrast, for the period as a whole, the spirits and wines sectors actually increased their employment of administrative, technical and clerical staff. Between 1963 and 1985 there was a general trend towards fewer operatives and relatively more administrative, technical and clerical workers,

Table 10.5

Number of operatives and administrative, clerical and technical employees, UK

Year	All Manufacturing (millions)		Tobacco		Brewing and Malting (thousands)		Spirits Distilling & Compounding		Wines, Cider and Perry	
	Opera-tives	Admin Tech and Clerical	Opera-tives	Admin Tech and Clerical	Opera-tives	Admin Tech and Clerical	Opera-tives	Admin Tech and Clerical	Opera-tives	Admin Tech and Clerical
1963	6.0	1.9	33.7	9.6	64.4	22.3	13.1	3.5	2.8	1.3
1970	5.9	2.1	29.1	10.6	51.8	22.7	17.3	4.9	3.7	1.5
1975	5.4	2.0	31.1	8.8	45.3	20.9	19.9	6.1	3.3	1.8
1980a	4.5	1.9	25.9	9.8	34.8	18.6	19.2	7.0	3.0	2.0
1984	3.4	1.6	17.9	8.9	24.9	12.7	12.2	5.5	2.6	2.1
1985	3.4	1.6	15.9	8.0	23.3	12.3	11.3	5.1	2.2	2.0
1986	n.a.	n.a.	13.5	7.0	22.8	12.5	11.1	5.0	2.2	1.9

a.   Introduction of 1980 SIC.

Source: *Census of Production,* Business Statistics Office, HMSO, London (annually).

thus resulting in a long-run decline in the ratio of operatives to other groups. Such trends are likely to be the result of new technology. In 1963, the ratio of operatives to other employees was 3.2 in manufacturing compared with 3.5 in tobacco and 2.9 in brewing. By 1985, the corresponding ratios were 2.1 in manufacturing, and under 2.0 in tobacco and brewing. On this basis, by 1985, brewing and tobacco were more skill-intensive than UK manufacturing.

Are the job losses amongst men or women and full- or part-time workers?

The tobacco industry is distinctive within manufacturing for employing a relatively high proportion of women. Table 10.6 shows that between 1971 and 1985, women accounted for some 70 per cent of total job losses in the tobacco industry, including a substantial *proportion* of part-time jobs. In contrast, during the same period, job losses in the alcohol industry appear to have been distributed equally between men and women.

Table 10.6

Male/female employment in tobacco and alcohol industries, GB

Year	Male	Numbers (thousands) Female		Per cent of total Male	Female
		Total	Part-time[b]	(%)	(%)
A. Tobacco industry					
1971	14.8	19.3	3.6	43.4	56.6
1975	15.0	19.0	3.2	44.1	55.9
1980	14.7	14.8	2.1	49.8	50.2
1985[a]	10.8	9.0	1.0	54.5	45.5
1986	9.2	7.6	0.7	54.8	45.2
B. Alcohol industry					
1971	75.7	25.1	3.0	75.1	24.9
1975	75.4	26.1	3.5	74.3	25.7
1980	73.3	25.2	3.3	74.4	25.6
1985	57.1	18.9	2.9	75.1	24.9
1986	56.0	18.5	2.8	75.2	24.8

a.   Introduction of the 1980 SIC.

b.   Working not more than 30 hours per week.

Source: Department of Employment, *Employment Gazette*, HMSO, London (annually).

For the tobacco industry, it is difficult to link the loss in female employment to the decline in cigarette consumption or to any particular government policy such as taxation. In terms of numbers of cigarettes, consumption levels peaked in 1973, after which they have declined being some 30 per cent lower in 1986 than at their peak (see Chapter 1, Table 1.6). However, the decline of the female labour force has been at a far faster rate, falling 60 per cent between 1975 and 1986 compared to a fall of 28 per cent in the number of cigarettes produced. This suggests that factors such as equal pay legislation and changes in technology in some parts of the manufacturing process may have altered the requirements for female labour, so leading to job losses. Questions then arise as to how far any technical change has been the direct or indirect result of actual and expected prevention policies.

Are job losses amongst the low-paid?

Any government concerned with equity and the distribution of income within society needs to know whether the job losses resulting from prevention policies are likely to be concentrated on the lower-paid and hence, poorer members of the community. Table 10.7 shows data on average wages and salaries in real terms. Between 1963 and 1985, all groups in brewing and tobacco had increased their incomes relative to UK manufacturing. Tobacco is especially interesting. After more than 20 years of prevention policies, operatives in particular have experienced a substantial improvement in their earnings position relative to all manufacturing. In other words, *future* job losses in tobacco are likely to involve workers with relatively high incomes. However, improvements in the relative pay of workers in tobacco (and brewing) are consistent with *past* job losses amongst the lower-paid. In this context, mention has already been made of job losses in tobacco concentrated amongst women, including part-time workers.

A paradox is apparent. The tobacco industry with declining domestic sales and a falling work-force, has experienced a substantial increase in the relative earnings of its employees. Higher wages could reflect new equipment and technology with an associated demand for a more skilled labour force; or they could reflect increased union bargaining power, especially if job losses have been borne largely by unorganised workers (e.g. women) with the unions obtaining a share in the industry's increased profitability (see Chapter 8). The interesting possibility arises that actual and expected prevention policies might have induced tobacco companies to adopt more efficient production processes, some of which have benefited their workers through higher incomes.

The location of job losses

Governments need to know the regional location of both job losses and of the remaining jobs in the alcohol and tobacco industries. Unfortunately, data on the geographical distribution of employment are limited to broad regions and do not provide a satisfactory time-series. Table 10.8 shows the regional distribution of employment in the tobacco and alcohol industries for Great Britain in 1984. Compared with all manufacturing, the tobacco industry is relatively concentrated in the South West, East Midlands, North and North West, with these regions accounting for 60 per cent of the industry's employment. Tobacco was also one of Northern Ireland's major manufacturing industries, although since 1985, a number of manufacturing plants have been closed (Scott, 1986, p.7). Brewing has an employment distribution similar to that of manufacturing, with some 50 per cent of its labour force in the Midlands, Yorkshire, North West and Scotland. Some

Table 10.7

Wages and salaries of operatives and administrative technical and clerical staff by industry, UK

	All Manufacturing	Tobacco	Brewing and Malting	Wines, Cider and Perry	Spirits, Distilling and
A. Operatives (£ per head per year, 1980 prices)					
1963	3234	2951	3459	2937	3078
1970	4032	3466	4574	3505	4188
1975	4613	5067	5689	4571	4683
1980a	4862	5687	6259	5807	4875
1984	5165	7608	6868	5553	5012
1985	5309	7866	6937	5677	5167
1986	n.a.	8281	7156	5646	5704
B. Administratives, technical and clerical (£ per head, 1980 prices)					
1963	4527	5068	4727	4502	5307
1970	5440	6029	5812	4747	6036
1975	6068	7413	5994	5178	6372
1980a	6351	7876	6693	5278	7084
1984	7054	10147	7826	7537	7699
1985	7249	10411	7700	8947	8161
1986	n.a.	11278	7864	8704	8554

a. Introduction of 1980 SIC figures adjusted to 1980 prices using all items Retail Price Index, average for the year.

Source: RPI figures from the Department of Employment, *Employment Gazette*, HMSO, London (monthly). Wages and salaries from Business Statistics Office, *Census of Production*, HMSO, London (annually).

limited data on employment trends in brewing between 1975 and 1984 showed that of some 17,000 job losses in Britain, over 50 per cent occurred in London, Yorkshire and the North West, with most of the remainder occurring in the North and West Midlands. Not surprisingly, spirits and distilling are concentrated in Scotland which accounted for some 80 per cent of the industry's employment in 1984 (see Chapter 9). Finally, the wines, cider and perry sector is heavily concentrated in the South West and the West Midlands. In aggregate, employment in the UK alcohol and tobacco industries is particularly concentrated in the South West, Midlands, North West, Scotland and Northern Ireland, which include some of the highest unemployment regions in the country.

Table 10.8

Regional distribution of employment 1984, G.B.[a]

Percentage of total (%)

Industry	Greater London	Rest of South East	East Anglia	South West	West Midlands	East Midlands	Yorkshire and Humberside	North West	North	Wales	Scotland
All industries and services	16.6	18.0	3.4	7.4	9.5	7.0	8.5	11.0	5.1	4.3	9.1
All manufacturing	10.7	17.2	3.6	7.1	13.3	9.2	9.1	12.6	5.2	4.0	8.1
Tobacco	18.6		3.0	19.1	-	16.4	0.7	16.7	8.7	4.0	9.4
Brewing and malting	15.7	11.8	4.6	6.6	15.1	5.4	9.1	13.9	6.8	3.3	8.1
Spirits	11.4	5.7	0.4	0.4	0.4	-	0.4	1.9	-	-	80.5
Wines, Cider and Perry	10.2	10.2	2.0	38.8	30.6	-	4.1	6.1	-	-.	-
Unemployment rate (%)	10.0	9.6	10.1	11.5	15.2	12.1	14.3	16.0	18.1	16.2	15.2

a. All data are for 1984 except for some of the tobacco, spirits and wines groups which are for 1981. These are the most recent data available.

Sources: Department of Employment, *Employment Gazette*, HMSO, London (monthly).

An indication is needed of the relative importance of employment in the alcohol and tobacco industries in each regions' economy. Given the broad geographical regions and the relatively small total work-force in these industries, it was not surprising to find that in most regions in Britain in 1981, the alcohol and tobacco industries each accounted for 0.5 per cent or less of all employment in each region. Scotland was an exception with the alcohol industry (spirits and distilling) accounting for 1.5 per cent of all jobs and some 6 per cent of manufacturing employment. This could partly explain why in the past, and potentially in the future, employment levels in Scotland might influence prevention policies aiming to reduce the consumption of spirits. However, the regional data are not sufficiently detailed to show the dependence of local communities on alcohol and tobacco plants.

As a limited exercise confined to tobacco, a geographical mapping was compiled of the industry's major plants in 1988. The results, based on press and trade sources, are shown in Table 10.9 which presents more detailed information on the regional distribution of employment. It can be seen that Bristol is the main location of tobacco plants in the South West, Nottingham for the East Midlands, Manchester and Liverpool in the North West, Darlington-Spennymoor in the North and Glasgow in Scotland (see Table 10.8). Since 1981, tobacco plants have been closed in Basildon, Bristol, Manchester, Nottingham, Newcastle, Glasgow, Stirling and in Northern Ireland. At the most, these plants and locations might be regarded as the losers from successive prevention policies (other things being equal). Many of the remaining tobacco plants are located in relatively high unemployment areas. It would be interesting to relate these locations to the political map, particularly to marginal constituencies.

CONCLUSION

This chapter has identified what is known and what is not known about the employment effects of prevention policies. Job losses in the alcohol and tobacco industries are not disputed. There are, though, genuine doubts about the magnitude of the employment losses and the extent to which they are attributable to prevention policies.

Direct job losses in the alcohol and tobacco industries have been relatively small. In the case of tobacco, direct job losses from *all causes* have been at an average rate of under 1,000 per annum. However, a substantial number of jobs are indirectly attributable to the alcohol and tobacco industries and are reflected in their backward and forward linkages from the raw materials through to the final consumer. The tobacco industry, for example, claims almost seven indirect jobs for every person employed

Table 10.9

Location of principal tobacco manufacturing plants, 1988

Company and Location	Size of Plant	Local Unemployment Rate (%)
Gallahers		
Belfast (due to close in 1988)	B	16.7
Lisnafillan	A	13.2
Hyde	A	11.8
Cardiff	B	11.6
Port Talbot	B	14.5
Imperial		
Bristol	A	8.1
Swindon (closed 1987)	C	7.3
Glasgow	A	15.9
Nottingham	A	10.8
Ipswich	B	5.4
Liverpool	C	18.5
Rothmans		
Darlington	B	12.3
Spennymoor	B	15.6
Peterlee	C	20.2
BAT (exports only)		
Liverpool	C	18.5
Southampton	B	8.1
Corby	C	10.9
Philip Morris		
London (Silvertown)	C	8.6

A = over 1000 employees; B = 500-1000 employees; C = under 500 employees.
Spennymoor and Peterlee are based on Stockton and Hartlepool, respectively; Hyde is based on Manchester.

Sources: Press reports and trade sources. Department of Employment, (1988), *Employment Gazette,* London, 96, (5), HMSO, London.

223

directly in the industry (Mackay and Edwards, 1982, p.16). Some of our own estimates of the ratio of indirect to direct jobs are much lower than the industry's figures. The various estimates are obviously sensitive to different assumptions, particularly in relation to employment in retailing.

Accepting that job losses in the alcohol and tobacco industries will have a 'knock-on' effect does not mean that all employment reductions have been caused by prevention policies. Employment can fall for a variety of reasons (for example, technology, changing competitiveness in both industry and retailing) of which prevention policies might be only one element. Nor does it follow that employment losses will be reflected in higher local unemployment. Much depends on the operation of local labour markets as reflected in the availability of other jobs, the willingness and ability of workers to move to different occupations and localities, and the willingness to work at various wage rates. It should also be stressed that effective prevention policies will release spending power for other purposes which will create new jobs. Such alternative spending is usually ignored. If prevention policies reduce the consumption of alcohol and tobacco, then consumers will search for alternative opportunities to spend their incomes and new patterns of spending will create new employment opportunities.

Questions remain. More information is required about the type of jobs which are indirectly due to alcohol and tobacco production. Do such workers have transferable skills which are likely to be valuable to large numbers of employers throughout the economy? Are the indirect workers men or women, full- or part-time and how much are they paid?

Some of the actual and potential losers from past and future prevention policies have been identified. Past losers have included operatives, women in the tobacco industry, together with plants located in high unemployment areas. In the future, potential losers are likely to be highly-paid. Such groups, although small in number but with more to lose, are likely to be even more hostile to prevention policies, and they will seek to influence government policy to favour their interests.

Notes

1. The authors are most grateful for comments from Larry Harrison, Alan Maynard, David Robinson and Philip Tether: the usual disclaimers apply.

2. The model was: $N = f(Q, t)$ where N = employment, Q = output and t = a time-trend representing technology. The equation was estimated in both linear and log-linear forms. An example for brewing and malting with all coefficients significant at the 1% level is: $N = 66.26 + 0.008Q - 2.45t$ ($R^2 = 0.99$; DW = 2.81; t = 1963–83 but missing observations for 1964–67 and 1969). See Hartley and Corcoran, 1975.

3. The model is derived from a general CES production function which allows for non-constant returns to scale. Employment is determined by output, the real wage rate, technology, capital and a lagged adjustment mechanism whereby actual employment adjusts to its desired level with a lag. This part of the empirical work was undertaken by Andrew Jones, Research Fellow, ARC, University of York.

References

Brewers Society, (1985), *Statistical Handbook*, Brewers Society, London.

Godfrey, C. and Hardman, G., (1987), 'Data Note 11, Employment in the UK alcohol and tobacco industries', *British Journal of Addiction*, 82, 1157–1167.

Godfrey, C. and Hartley, K., (1988), 'Data Note 16, Employment and prevention policy', *British Journal of Addiction*, 83, 1335–1342.

Hartley, K. and Corcoran, W., (1975), 'Short-run employment functions and defence contracts in the UK aircraft industry', *Applied Economics*, 7, 223–233.

Mackay, D., (1985), *The Tobacco Industry in the European Community Including Portugal and Spain*, Peida, Edinburgh.

Mackay, D.I. and Edwards, R.T., (1982), *The UK Tobacco Industry: Its Economic Significance*, Peida, Edinburgh.

Scott, M., (1986), *The Economic Consequences of Smoking in Northern Ireland*, Ulster Cancer Foundation, Belfast.

Tobacco Advisory Council, (1985), 'Why unfair tobacco taxation makes the dole queue longer, advertisement', *The Times*, Friday, March 5th, 6.

Contents of Volume 2:

Manipulating Consumption: information, law and voluntary controls

Foreword

Editors' introduction:
Christine Godfrey and David Robinson

Chapter 1: Regulation
Larry Harrison, Philip Tether and Rob Baggott

Chapter 2: Information and voluntary agreements: the policy networks
Larry Harrison and Philip Tether

Chapter 3: Alcohol advertising
Larry Harrison and Christine Godfrey

Chapter 4: Tobacco advertising
Philip Tether and Christine Godfrey

Chapter 5: Legislation: the policy networks
Philip Tether, Wendy Leedham and Larry Harrison

Chapter 6: Liquor licensing
Philip Tether and Christine Godfrey

Chapter 7: Drinking and driving
Philip Tether and Christine Godfrey

Chapter 8: Preventing alcohol and tobacco problems
Alan Maynard and David Robinson

Addiction Research Centre bibliography

Alaszewski, A. and Harrison, L., (1989), 'Collaboration and coordination between welfare agencies', *British Journal of Social Work*, (forthcoming).

Anderson, P., Bennison, J., Orford, J., Spratley, T., Tether, P., Tomson, J. and Wilson, T., (1986), *Alcohol: A Balanced View*, Report from General Practice No. 24, Royal College of General Practitioners, London.

Baggott, R., (1986), 'By voluntary agreement: the politics of instrument selection', *Public Administration*, 64, 51–68.

Baggott, R., (1986), 'Alcohol, politics and social policy', *Journal of Social Policy*, 15, 467–488.

Baggott, R., (1986), *The Politics of Alcohol: Two Periods Compared*, Occasional Paper No. 8, Institute of Alcohol Studies, London.

Baggott, R., (1987), 'Government Industry Relations in Britain: the regulation of the tobacco industry', *Policy and Politics*, 15, 3, 137–146.

Baggott, R., (1987), *Licensing Law Reform: Social Welfare or Public Thirst*, Occasional Paper No. 12, Institute for Alcohol Studies, London.

Baggott, R., (1987), *The Politics of Public Health: Alcohol, Politics and Social Policy*, Ph.D. Thesis, University of Hull.

Baggott, R., (1988), 'Drinking and driving: the politics of social regulation', *Teaching Politics*, 17, 66–85.

Baggott, R., (1988), *Health v Wealth: The Politics of Smoking in Norway and the UK*, Papers on Government and Politics No. 57, University of Strathclyde, Glasgow.

Baggott, R., (1988), 'Licensing law reform and the return of the drink question', *Parliamentary Affairs*.

Baggott, R., (1989), 'Alcohol and tobacco: the politics of prevention', in Maynard, A. and Tether, P. (eds.), *The Addiction Market: consumption, production and policy development*, Avebury/Gower, Aldershot.

Baggott, R., (1989), 'The politics of the market', in Robinson, D., Maynard, A. and Chester, R. (eds.), *Controlling Legal Addictions*, Macmillan, London.

229

Baggott, R. and Harrison, L., (1986), 'The politics of self regulation: the case of advertising control', *Policy and Politics*, 14, 143–159.

Booth, M., Hardman, G. and Hartley, K., (1986), 'Data Note 6, The UK alcohol and tobacco industries', *British Journal of Addiction*, 81, 825–830.

Booth, M., Hardman, G. and Hartley, K., (1988), 'Data Note 14, Mergers in the UK alcohol and tobacco industries', *British Journal of Addiction*, 83, 707–714.

Booth, M., Hartley, K. and Powell, M., (1989), 'Industry and employment policy: department and group relations', in Maynard, A. and Tether P. (eds.), *The Addiction market: consumption, production and policy development*, Avebury/Gower, Aldershot.

Booth, M. and Weir, R., (1989), 'Prevention and policy in the Scotch whisky industry', in Maynard, A. and Tether, P., (eds.), *The Addiction Market: consumption, production and policy development*, Avebury/Gower, Aldershot.

Godfrey, C., (1986), Factors Influencing the Consumption of Alcohol and Tobacco—A Review of Demand Models, Discussion Paper 17, Centre for Health Economics, University of York.

Godfrey, C., (1986), 'Government policy, advertising and tobacco consumption in the UK: a critical review of the literature', *British Journal of Addiction*, 81, 339–346.

Godfrey, C., (1988), 'Licensing and the demand for alcohol', *Applied Economics*, 20, 1541–1558.

Godfrey, C., (1989), 'Modelling demand', in Maynard, A. and Tether, P. (eds.), *The Addiction Market: consumption, production and policy development*, Avebury/Gower, Aldershot.

Godfrey, C., (1989), 'Evaluating alternative advertising policies', in *Alcohol Advertising: Who Benefits? Why Ban?*, Action and Alcohol Abuse, London.

Godfrey, C., (1989), 'Price regulation', in Robinson, D., Maynard, A. and Chester, R. (eds.), *Controlling Legal Addictions*, Macmillan, London.

Godfrey, C., (1989), 'Factors influencing the consumption of alcohol: the use and abuse of economic models', *British Journal of Addiction*, (forthcoming).

Godfrey, C. and Hardman, G., (1987), 'Data note 11, Employment in the UK alcohol and tobacco industries', *British Journal of Addiction*, 82, 1157–1167.

Godfrey, C., Hardman, G. and Maynard, A., (1986), 'Data Note 2, Measuring UK alcohol consumption', *British Journal of Addiction*, 81, 287–293.

Godfrey, C., Hardman, G. and Powell, M., (1986), 'Data Note 1, Alcohol, tobacco and taxation', *British Journal of Addiction*, 81, 143–149.

Godfrey, C. and Harrison, L., (1989), 'Alternative tax policies', in Maynard, A. and Tether, P. (eds.), *The Addiction Market: consumption, production and policy development*, Avebury/Gower, Aldershot.

Godfrey, C. and Hartley, K., (1988), 'Data Note 16, Employment and prevention policy', *British Journal of Addiction*, 83, 1335–1342.

Godfrey, C. and Hartley, K., (1989), 'Employment', in Maynard, A. and Tether, P. (eds.), *The Addiction Market: consumption, production and policy development*, Avebury/Gower, Aldershot.

Godfrey, C. and Maynard, A., (1988), 'Economic aspects of tobacco use and taxation policy', *British Medical Journal*, 297, 339–343.

Godfrey, C. and Maynard, A., (1988), 'An economic theory of alcohol consumption and abuse', in Chaudron, D. and Wilkinson, A. (eds.), *Theories of Alcoholism*, Addiction Research Foundation, Toronto.

Godfrey, C. and Powell, M., (1986), 'Alcohol and tobacco taxation: barriers to a public health perspective', *Quarterly Journal of Social Affairs*, 1, 329–252.

Godfrey, C. and Powell, M., (1987), Budget Strategies for Alcohol and Tobacco in 1987 and Beyond, Discussion Paper 22, Centre for Health Economics, University of York.

Godfrey, C. and Powell, M., (1987), 'Making sense of the social cost studies of alcohol, drugs and tobacco', in *The Cost of Alcohol, Drugs and Tobacco to Society*, 31–52, Institute for Preventive and Social Psychiatry, Erasmus University, Rotterdam.

Godfrey, C. and Powell, M., (1989), 'The relationship between Government policy and individual choice in the decision to consume hazardous goods', in Baldwin, S., Godfrey, C. and Propper, C. (eds.), *Quality of Life: Policy and Perspectives*, Routledge, London.

Godfrey, C. and Robinson, D. (eds.), (1989), *Manipulating Consumption: information, law and voluntary controls*, Avebury/Gower, Aldershot.

Hardman, G. and Maynard, A., (1989), 'Consumption and taxation', in Maynard, A. and Tether, P. (eds.), *The Addiction Market: consumption, production and policy development, Avebury/Gower, Aldershot.*

Harrison, L., (1985), 'Light the blue touch-paper: the cigarette as a fire hazard', *Radical Community Medicine*, 27–28.

Harrison, L., (1986), 'Is a coordinated prevention policy really feasible?', *Alcohol and Alcoholism*, 21, 5–6.

Harrison, L., (1986), 'Tobacco battered and the pipes shattered; a note on the fate of the first British campaign against tobacco smoking', *British Journal of Addiction*, 81, 553–558.

Harrison, L., (1987), 'Data Note 7, Drinking and driving in Great Britain', *British Journal of Addiction*, 82, 203–208.

Harrison, L., (1987), 'Drinking and driving in Northern Ireland', *British Journal of Addiction*, 82, 210.

Harrison, L., (1988), 'Alcohol statistics: time to sort out the muddle', *Alliance News*, 14–16.

Harrison, L., (1988), 'The deadly habit that Governments can't give up', *The Listener*, 21 January, 15.

Harrison, L., (1989), 'Research perspectives, 2', in Steele, D. (ed.), *Alcohol Advertising: Who Benefits Why Ban?*, Action on Alcohol Abuse, London.

Harrison, L., (1989), 'The information component', in Robinson, D., Maynard, A., and Chester, R. (eds.), *Controlling Legal Addictions*, Macmillan, London.

Harrison, L. and Godfrey, C., (1989), 'Alcohol advertising', in Godfrey, C. and Robinson, D. (eds.), *Manipulating Consumption: information, law and voluntary controls*, Avebury/Gower, Aldershot.

Harrison, L. and Godfrey, C., (1989), 'Alcohol advertising controls in the 1990s', *International Journal of Advertising*, (forthcoming).

Harrison, L. and Tether, P., (1987), 'Coordinating the UK's policy on alcohol and tobacco: the significance of organisational networks', *Policy and Politics*, 15, 77–90.

Harrison, L. and Tether, P., (1988), 'Data Note 13, Alcohol policy and the British Government bureaucracy', *British Journal of Addiction*, 83, 451–460.

Harrison, L. and Tether, P., (1989), 'Tax policy: structure and process', in Maynard, A. and Tether, P. (eds.), *The Addiction Market: consumption, production and policy development*, Avebury/Gower, Aldershot.

231

Harrison, L. and Tether, P., (1989), 'Information and voluntary agreements: the policy networks', in Godfrey, C. and Robinson, D. (eds.), *Manipulating Consumption: information, law and voluntary controls*, Avebury/Gower, Aldershot.

Harrison, L., Tether, P. and Baggott, R., (1989), 'Regulation and voluntary agreements', in Godfrey, C. and Robinson, D. (eds.), *Manipulating Consumption: information, law and voluntary controls*, Avebury/Gower, Aldershot.

Hartley, K., (1985), 'Exogenous factors in economic theory: neoclassical economics', *Social Science Information*, 24, 457–483.

Hartley, K., (1985), 'Bureaucracy and power without responsibility', *Economic Affairs*, 6, 16–18.

Hartley, K., (1989), 'Industry, employment and prevention policy', in Robinson, D., Maynard, A. and Chester, R. (eds.), *Controlling Legal Addictions*, Macmillan, London.

Hartley, K., (1989), 'Alcohol, tobacco and public policy: the contribution of economics', *British Journal of Addiction*, (forthcoming).

Jones, A., (1986), First Hurdle Dominance: Theoretical Foundations for an Empirical Investigation of Cigarette Consumption, Discussion Paper 117, Department of Economics, University of York.

Jones, A., (1987), *A Theoretical and Empirical Investigation of the Demand for Addictive Goods*, D.Phil Thesis, University of York.

Jones, A., (1987), A Double-Hurdle Model of Cigarette Consumption, Discussion Paper 128, Department of Economics, University of York.

Jones, A., (1989), 'The UK demand for cigarettes 1954–1986, a double-hurdle approach', *Journal of Health Economics*, (forthcoming).

Jones, A. and Posnett, J., (1988), 'The revenue and welfare effects of cigarette taxes', *Applied Economics*, 20, 1223–1232.

Keeley Robinson, Y. and Baggott, R., (1985), 'Health education and the prevention of alcohol-related problems', *Health Education Journal*, 44, 174–177.

Leedham, W., (1987), 'Data Note 10, Alcohol, tobacco and public opinion', *British Journal of Addiction*, 82, 935–940.

Leedham, W. and Godfrey, C., (1989), 'Tax policy and budget decisions', in Maynard, A. and Tether, P. (eds.), *The Addiction Market: consumption, production and policy development*, Avebury/Gower, Aldershot.

Maynard, A., (1983), 'Modelling alcohol consumption and abuse', in Grant, M., Plant, M. and Williams, A. (eds.), *Economics and Alcohol*, Croom Helm, London.

Maynard, A., (1984), 'The social costs of alcohol use', in *Alcohol: Preventing the Harm*, Conference proceedings published by the Institute of Alcohol Studies, 232–242.

Maynard, A., (1985), 'The role of economic measures in preventing drinking problems', in Heather, N., Robertson, I. and Davies, P. (eds.), *The Misuse of Alcohol*, Croom Helm, London.

Maynard, A., (1985), 'Alcohol: preventing the harm', *Alliance News*, 3693, 3–4.

Maynard, A., (1985), 'Alcohol use: costs and benefits', *Alcohol Concern*, 11–12.

Maynard, A., (1986), 'Economic aspects of addiction policy', *Health Promotion Journal*, 1, 61–71.

Maynard, A., (1987), 'A economia das toxico-dependencias', in Correlade Campos, A. and Pereira, J.A. (eds.), *Sociedade, Sande e Economia*, Escola Nacional De Saude Publica, Lisbon.

Maynard, A., (1989), 'Price as a determinant of alcohol consumption', *Australian Drug and Alcohol Review*, (forthcoming).

Maynard, A., (1989), 'The costs of addiction and the costs of control', in Robinson, D., Maynard, A. and Chester, R. (eds.), *Controlling Legal Addictions*, Macmillan, London.

Maynard, A., Hardman, G. and Whelan, A., (1987), 'Data Note 9, Measuring the social costs of addictive substances', *British Journal of Addiction/, 82, 701–706.*

Maynard, A. and Jones, A., (1987), *Economic Aspects of Addiction Control Policies*, Centre for Health Economics and Addiction Research Centre, University of York.

Maynard, A. and O'Brien, B., (1982), 'Harmonisation policies in the European Community and alcohol abuse', *British Journal of Addiction*, 77, 235–244.

Maynard, A. and Powell, M., (1985), 'Addiction control policies, or there's no such thing as a free lunch', *British Journal of Addiction*, 80, 265–267.

Maynard, A. and Robinson, D., (1989), 'Preventing alcohol and tobacco problems', in Godfrey, C. and Robinson, D. (eds.), *Manipulating Consumption: information, law and voluntary controls*, Avebury/Gower, Aldershot.

Maynard, A. and Tether, P. (eds.), (1989), *The Addiction Market: consumption, production and policy development*, Avebury/Gower, Aldershot.

McDonnell, R. and Maynard, A., (1985), 'The costs of alcohol misuse', *British Journal of Addiction*, 80, 27–35.

McDonnell, R. and Maynard, A., (1985), 'Counting the costs of alcohol: gaps in epidemiological knowledge', *Community Medicine*, 7, 4–17.

McDonnell, R. and Maynard, A., (1985), 'Estimation of life years lost from alcohol-related premature death', *Alcohol and Alcoholism*, 20, 435–443.

Powell, M., (1987), 'Data Note 8, Alcohol data in the European Community', *British Journal of Addiction*, 82, 559–566.

Powell, M., (1988), 'Data Note 15, Alcohol and tobacco tax in the European Community', *British Journal of Addiction*, 83, 971–978.

Powell, M., (1988), 'Licence reform: less regulation, more individual restraint?', *Contemporary Review*, 253 (1474), 243–247.

Powell, M., (1989), 'UK opposition to tobacco tax harmonisation: the hidden agenda', *Contemporary Review*, 254 (1477), 77–82.

Powell, M., (1989), 'Behind the smoke screen: a data analysis of the tobacco industry', *Business Studies*, (forthcoming).

Powell, M., (1989), *Economic Aspects of Alcohol Policy: Prevention or Profits*, Routledge, (forthcoming).

Powell, M., (1989), 'Tax harmonisation in the EC', in Robinson, D., Maynard, A. and Chester, R. (eds.), *Controlling Legal Addictions*, Macmillan, London.

Powell, M., (1989), 'The health policy implications of international trade in alcohol and tobacco', *British Journal of Addiction*, (forthcoming).

Robinson, D., (1983), 'SSRC Addiction Research Centre', *British Journal of Addiction*, 78, 227–229.

Robinson, D., (1983), 'The growth of Alcoholics Anonymous', *Alcohol and Alcoholism*, 18, 167–172.

Robinson, D., (1985), 'The WHO three-centre study: a good first step', *British Journal of Addiction*, 80, 137.

Robinson, D., (1986), 'Data for informed debate', *British Journal of Addiction*, 81, 6.

Robinson, D., (1986), 'Mutual aid in the change process', in Heather, B. and Miller, P. (eds.), *Treating Addictive Behaviours*, Plenum, New York.

Robinson, D., (1986), 'Alcohol, education and action: shifting emphases', *Health Education Research: Theory and Practice*, 1, 325– 331.

Robinson, D., (1987), *Preventing Alcohol Problems*, the first Aquarius lecture, Aquarius, Birmingham.

Robinson, D., (1988), 'Prevention policy: alcohol and tobacco', *ESRC Newsletter*, 62, 12–14.

Robinson, D., (1989), 'Controlling legal addictions: taking advantage of what's there', in Robinson, D., Maynard, A. and Chester, R. (eds.), *Controlling Legal Addictions*, Macmillan, London.

Robinson, D. and Maynard, A., (1987), 'Reports from research centres – 5, Addiction Research Centre: Hull-York, UK', *British Journal of Addiction*, 82, 1185–1190.

Robinson, D. and Maynard, A., (1989), *Alcohol: Preventing a Legal Addiction*, ESRC Briefing, (forthcoming).

Robinson, D., Maynard, A. and Chester, R.L.C. (eds.), (1989), *Controlling Legal Addictions*, Macmillan, London.

Robinson, D. and Maynard, A., (1989), 'Controlling legal addictions', *British Journal of Addiction*, (forthcoming).

Robinson, D. and Tether, P., (1983), 'The environment debate', in Grant, M. and Ritson, B. (eds.), *Alcohol: the Prevention Debate*, Croom Helm, London.

Robinson, D. and Tether, P., (1985), 'Prevention: potential at the local level', *Alcohol and Alcoholism*, 20, 31–33.

Robinson, D. and Tether, P., (1987), 'Alcohol problems: (i) prevention at the local level', *Health Trends*, 19, 19–22.

Robinson, D. and Tether, P., (1989), *Preventing Alcohol Problems: Local Prevention Activity and the Compilation of 'Guides to Local Action'*, World Health Organisation, Geneva, (forthcoming).

Robinson, D., Tether, P. and Teller, J. (eds.), (1989), *Local Action on Alcohol Problems*, Routledge, London, (forthcoming).

Tether, P., (1985), *Preventing Alcohol-Related Accidents: A Guide to Local Action*, Occasional Paper No. 6, Institute of Alcohol Studies, London.

Tether, P., (1985), 'A lethal cocktail: alcohol and water', *Alcohol Concern*, 1, 13–14.

Tether, P., (1986), 'Cutting the risks of alcohol at sea', *Alcohol Concern*, 2, 6–8.

Tether, P., (1987), 'Preventing alcohol-related problems: the local dimension', in Stockwell, T. and Clement, S. (eds.), *Helping the Problem Drinker*, Croom Helm, London.

Tether, P., (1989), 'Legal controls and voluntary agreements', in Robinson, D., Maynard, A. and Chester, R. (eds.), *Controlling Legal Addictions*, Macmillan, London.

Tether, P. and Godfrey, C., (1989), 'Tobacco advertising', in Godfrey, C. and Robinson, D. (eds.), *Manipulating Consumption: information, law and voluntary controls*, Avebury/Gower, Aldershot.

Tether, P. and Godfrey, C., (1989), 'Liquor licensing', in Godfrey, C. and Robinson, D. (eds.), *Manipulating Consumption: information, law and voluntary controls*, Avebury/Gower, Aldershot.

Tether, P. and Godfrey, C., (1989), 'Drinking and driving', in Godfrey, C. and Robinson, D. (eds.), *Manipulating Consumption: information, law and voluntary controls*, Avebury/Gower, Aldershot.

Tether, P. and Harrison, L., (1986), 'Data Note 3, Alcohol-related fires and drowning', *British Journal of Addiction*, 81, 425–431.

Tether, P. and Harrison, L., (1988), *Alcohol Policies: Responsibilities and Relationship in British Government*, Addiction Research Centre, Universities of Hull and York.

Tether, P. and Harrison, L., (1989), 'Industry and employment policy: department and group relations', in Maynard, A. and Tether, P. (eds.), *The Addiction Market: consumption, production and policy development*, Avebury/Gower, Aldershot.

Tether, P., Leedham, W. and Harrison, L., (1989), 'Legislation: the policy networks', in Godfrey, C. and Robinson, D. (eds.), *Manipulating Consumption: information, law and voluntary controls*, Avebury/Gower, Aldershot.

Tether, P. and Robinson, D., (1985), 'Alcohol and work: 'policies' are not enough', *Alcohol and Alcoholism*, 20, 1–3.

Tether, P. and Robinson, D., (1986), *Preventing Alcohol Problems: A Guide to Local Action*, Tavistock Publications, London.

Tether, P. and Robinson, D., (1988), 'Alcohol problems: (ii) alcohol and work', *Health Trends*, 20, 24–26.

Tether, P., Robinson, D. and Wicks, M., (1984), 'Liquor licensing: its role in a prevention strategy', *Alcohol and Alcoholism*, 19, 272– 79.

Wagstaff, A. and Maynard, A., (1986), 'Data Note 5, The consumption of illicit drugs in the UK', *British Journal of Addiction*, 81, 691– 696.

Wagstaff, A. and Maynard, A., (1988), *Economic Aspects of the Illicit Drug Market and Drug Enforcement Policies in the United Kingdom*, Home Office Research Study No. 95, HMSO, London.

Weir, R., (1984), 'Distilling and agriculture 1870–1939', *The Agricultural History Review*, 32, 20–33.

Weir, R., (1984), 'Obsessed with moderation: the drink trades and the drink question', *British Journal of Addiction*, 79, 93–107.

Weir, R., (1988), 'Alcohol controls and Scotch whisky exports 1900– 1939', *British Journal of Addiction*, 83, 1289–1297.

Index

AAA *see* Alcohol Abuse
ADD *see* Ministry of Agriculture, Fisheries and Food. Alcoholic Drinks Division
ARC *see* Addiction Research Centre
ASA *see* Advertising Standards Authority
ASH *see* Action on Smoking and Health
absenteeism 144, 148
accidents 8
Action on Alcohol Abuse (AAA) 64, 88, 100, 118, 127, 141
Action on Smoking and Health (ASH) 4, 88, 97, 98, 100, 118, 127
addiction market 4, 6, 7
Addiction Research Centre xii, xiv, 6, 198
addictive substances 3, 155
administration 78, 81, 84; Conservative 96, 97; costs 61, 66, 68
administrative constraints model *see* models
administrative procedures 77
administrative processes 76
administrative services 85
administrative structures 76, 77
administrative theories 78
administrative units 93, 137

administrators 80, 90, 91
Adjournment Debates *see* Parliamentary procedures
ad valorem taxes *see* tax ad valorem
advertisers 146
advertising xiv, 36, 39, 119, 124, 137, 153–155 *passim*, 171, 174, 176, 208
—agencies 205
—alcohol 154
—ban on 46, 51, 119–121 *passim*, 129, 158, 171, 205
—cigarette 46, 119, 121, 174, 205
—codes of practice 145
—control of 158, 176, 208
—drinks 125
—effects (general) 37–38, 47
—effects on tobacco consumption 35, 45–51 *passim*
—expenditure on 37
—industry 125, 145, 151, 204
—on TV 46, 119, 121, 125, 129, 171
—poster 125
—revenue from 125, 129
—tobacco 145
Advertising Standards Authority (ASA) 145
agriculture 200, 201, 210
—farmers 125, 135

—farming interests 148
alcohol 8–10, 14, 19, 42, 48–50, 62, 65,
68, 72, 75, 76, 82, 117, 118, 121, 126
—abuse 38, 119, 120, 126, 130; health
consequences, implications of abuse
97, 99, 124, 147; problems of abuse
83, 103, 117, 122, 125, 128, 129,
137, 142; and young people 67, 127,
128
—availability of 119, 171, 176
—consumption 1, 2, 8, 9, 12, 15, 32,
35–43 passim, 50, 59, 75, 82, 83, 93,
100, 109, 115, 126, 129, 152, 180,
212; benefits of reducing
consumption 179; increase in
consumption 15, 32, 99; reduction in
consumption 65, 100, 122, 146, 179,
224; per capita intake 15, 100, 139,
179; trends in consumption 83
—demand for 35, 36, 39, 44, 176, 179,
215
—duty rates 29, 58, 65, 76, 77, 83, 86,
89, 91, 92, 93, 100, 109, 111, 113,
114, 140; revenue from duty 103, 113
—economic role of alcohol 102
—expenditure 9, 11
—importers 139, 140
—industry 1, 5, 6, 8, 12, 82–89 passim,
100-102, 118–132 passim, 133–150
passim, 151–179 passim, 187, 204,
207–225 passim; employment 210,
215
—issues 120, 121, 124, 126, 127, 143
—policy 82, 119, 121, 134, 137, 147
—price of 54, 63, 66, 86, 93, 99, 109
—pure alcohol 14, 15, 36, 56
—tax policy 54–74, 104
—taxation 4, 26, 30, 31, 32, 58–61, 67,
69, 71, 72, 76, 82, 96, 97, 101–108
passim, 115, 122, 129, 179; changes
in 97; per cent alcohol 67; per unit
alcohol 67; per volume 2, 27, 56, 113
—trade 71, 100–102, 139; agricultural
side 88; markets and marketing 1, 2,
11, 83, 125, 151, 152, 154, 159;
production and producers 6, 88, 118,
134, 138–144 passim, 149, 154, 212;
production policy 5, 119, 123, 128,
135, 138, 139, 146, 173; products 2,

151, 152, 177, 205; sales 5, 6, 204;
wholesale and distribution trades 143
—use xiii, 3, 4, 7, 9, 124
—voluntary alcohol services 119
Alcohol Concern 61, 65, 100, 127, 133,
146
alcohol policy coordinator 148
Alcohol Studies, Institute for see
Institute for Alcohol Studies
alcoholic content 15, 100, 139
alcoholic drinks 9, 10, 11, 12, 70, 85,
92, 157, 159, 199
—consumption of 12, 14
—duties on 84
—expenditure on 2, 11, 13, 32, 125
—low alcoholic drinks 67
—market for 6, 11, 12
—taxation on 75, 100
—trade in 139
—beer 9–19, 42, 43, 48, 49, 60, 62, 68,
108, 110, 112, 125, 139, 144, 155,
159, 160, 162, 166, 199;
consumption 12, 13, 43, 50, 69;
demand 38; draught beer 22, 23, 24,
25, 156; duty on 84, 85, 109, 113;
expenditure on 11, 32, 49; industry
71; lager 9, 139, 156, 159; prices 2,
19, 20–22, 32, 37, 63, 66, 106, 107,
109; production 84; taxation of 27,
28, 58, 65, 66, 67, 105, 106
—cider 10–19 passim, 110, 112, 125,
139, 156, 157, 159, 160, 209, 217,
220; consumption of 12; expenditure
on 11, 32; price of 19, 21, 106;
production 84; sales 13; taxation 29,
67, 106
—perry 10, 11, 12, 19, 156, 157, 159,
160, 209, 217, 220; expenditure on
11, 32; price 19
—spirits 1, 10–19 passim, 42, 43, 48,
49, 60, 62, 68, 106, 108, 110, 112,
125, 144, 156, 159–165 passim, 187,
199, 201; consumption of 2, 12, 13,
37, 48, 50, 69, 182, 184, 187, 202,
222; demand for 40; employment
levels 210; expenditure on 11, 32, 48;
gin 139, 156, 182, 184, 194; industry
71, 115, 125, 216, 220, 220; prices 2,
19, 21, 32, 63, 65, 106; production

84, 159; sales 13; taxation 29, 56, 58, 65, 68, 69, 105, 106, 111; vodka 139, 156, 194; warehousing 84
—whisky 6, 21, 101, 110, 112, 156, 179–203; blended 181, 182, 183, 190, 196; consumption of 6, 183, 190, 194, 199; demand for 181, 191, 194, 198, 200, 202; exports 195; grain 180, 181, 190; malt 180, 181, 196; prices 6, 21, 23, 67, 107, 182; production 190; sales 187, 290; Scotch 139, 140, 179-203; taxation of 182, 198
—wine 1, 10–19 *passim*, 27, 42, 48, 49, 60, 62, 68, 108, 110, 112, 125, 139, 144, 156, 157, 159–165 *passim*, 187, 199; British wine/sherry 139, 199; consumption of 2, 12, 32, 43, 48, 50, 69; expenditure on 11, 32, 48; industry (including English wine industry) 139, 209, 216, 217, 220; employment levels in wine industry 210; prices 2, 19, 21, 24, 32, 63, 106; production 84; sales 13; taxation and duties 26, 27, 29–30, 32, 65, 66, 67, 69, 106; trade 139; warehousing 84
All Party Group for Action on Smoking and Health 98
All Party Group on Scotch Whisky 118
Allied Lyons 160, 162, 163, 167, 169, 186
anti-alcohol campaigns 127, 182, 183
anti-smoking campaigns 120, 127, 159
anti-smoking groups 97
anti-smoking policies 126
Argyll 186, 187–188
Arthur Bell and Sons 183, 185, 186
Autumn Statement *see* Budget

BMA *see* British Medical Association
balance of payments 82, 83
balance of trade *see* trade, balance of
bargaining 77, 79, 87, 93
Bass 162, 163, 167, 169, 174, 185
beer *see* alcoholic drinks
benchmark policies 3, 61, 65–66, 113
black market 155, 190
blending 182, 186, 193
bottling 182, 192, 193, 196

breathalyser 199, 129
broking 182, 193
brewers 2, 5, 85, 101, 121, 125, 126, 140, 154–174 *passim*, 185; financial contributions to political parties 121; suppliers to 143
Brewers Society 118, 124, 125, 176
brewing 6, 156, 157, 160, 164, 165, 169, 174, 177, 183, 201, 207, 209, 210; industry 156, 159, 162, 165, 166, 177, 172, 175, 200, 207, 213, 214, 216, 219, 220
British American Tobacco (BAT) 162, 163, 165, 167, 168, 169
British Medical Association (BMA) 98, 126, 127, 128, 141
British Retailers Association 88, 124–125
Budget, the 28, 63, 65, 67, 75–95 *passim*, 97, 100, 104, 108, 109, 111;
—Annual Budget Statement 97, 106, 107, 109;
—Autumn Statement 87, 88;
—Budget Green Paper 87;
—departmental 90;
—"mini Budget" 108;
—pre-Budget discussions 100, 143;
—pre-Budget submissions 100, 102
budget calculations 140
budget changes 106
budget decisions 72, 76, 78, 92, 96–116
budget policy 4, 63, 98, 101–116
budget proposals 62
budget surveys 41
budgetary adjustments 61–66
budgetary options 84
budgetary process 77, 87, 90, 92, 96, 101
budgetary system 54
bureaucratic organisations 77, 80
bureaucratic politics 77–80, 90, 92
bureaucrats 78, 79

Cabinet 79, 81, 88, 89, 90, 119, 122, 136, 137
Cabinet committees 81, 137
Campaign for Real Ale (CAMRA) 125, 141
Castle, Barbara 119, 136
Chancellor of the Exchequer 4, 59, 62,

63, 71, 75–95 *passim*, 96–116
passim; Conservative 4; Labour 4
children
—protection of 57
—and alcohol 127
Churches Council on Alcohol and Drugs
(CCAD) 127
cider *see* alcoholic drinks
cigarettes 9, 15, 17, 18, 28, 36, 42, 62,
99, 110, 112, 155, 156, 162
—brands 9, 174; companies 154;
consumption of 15, 18, 26, 43, 45, 69,
218; demand for 39, 40, 42; duty on
86; exports 170; filter 15, 25, 56;
high tar 36, 56, 68, 109; low tar 15,
36, 56; number smoked 56; plain 15,
56; price of 21, 25, 40, 63, 65, 104,
106, 107, 109; production of 210;
sales of 15, 98, 170, 215; smoking of
18; tar content of 85, 156; taxes on
26, 63, 66, 69, 75, 104, 106, 113,
129, 205
cigarillos 15, 17
cigars 15, 17, 28, 42, 113, 156
—consumption of 69
civil servants 90, 121, 78, 79, 81, 83,
87, 91, 92, 92, 122, 137
Civil Service 121, 82, 90
clubs 151, 164, 175, 211, 212
companies 172, 177
—alcohol 161, 163, 169, 174, 188, 189
—brewing 167, 168, 176, 183, 186
—cigarette 176
—distilling 168
—foreign 175
—multinational 162, 187
—tobacco 5, 161–176 *passim*, 188
—whisky 186, 189, 195
company decisions 168
company ownership 166–169
company performance *see* industry
performance
competition 39, 93, 153, 158, 161, 164,
165, 174, 175, 185, 187, 202
competition policy 143, 174, 175 *see
also* models, perfect competition
competitive markets 173
competitiveness 166, 210, 224
compounding 156, 194, 199, 209, 217

Conservative Party 4, 115, 121, 123, 147
—manifesto 120; policies 97
Conservative Women's National
Committee 98
consumer expenditure 124, 159
consumer goods and services 141
consumer interests 102, 135, 148; safety
interests 144, 148
consumer organisations 125
consumer preferences (tastes) 165, 173,
187, 199
consumers 1, 7, 41, 57–59 *passim*,
151–155 *passim*, 174, 176, 177, 183,
204, 205, 210, 215, 216, 222, 224
—and choice 60, 173, 177
consumption 1, 6, 8, 9, 14, 17, 18, 19,
56, 57, 60, 62, 128, 148, 151, 155,
205, 215
—at home 14
—control of 54, 103, 105, 115
—effects of 69
—habits 109
—harmful aspects of 36, 55, 56
—levels of 41, 43, 47–49 *passim*, 54,
56, 218
—measures used 9, 36–37
—patterns of 1, 8, 11, 15, 19, 71, 216
—per capita 57, 65
—policy 2, 7, 57
—reduction in 176, 207, 208
—trends 1, 2, 6, 8, 43, 62, 64, 65
—variations in 8, 43, 62, 64, 65
—volume 2, 9, 12–19, 33; *see also*
tobacco consumption; *see also*
alcohol consumption
control policy 5, 100, 104, 105, 177
controls 6
—legal xiv, 145, 147
—voluntary xiv
corporations *see* companies
cost-benefit analysis 143
costs 1, 55, 56, 143
—increases in 66
—manufacturers' 62, 63, 64
—transportation 71;
see also administration costs;
see also social costs
Courage 156, 161, 162, 165
Customs and Excise *see* HM Customs

and Excise
customs duty *see* tax

DCL *see* Distillers Co.
DHSS *see* Department of Health and
  Social Security
DPU *see* HM Customs and Excise.
  Departmental Planning Unit
DTI *see* Department of Trade and
  Industry
decision makers 89
decision making 1, 78, 87, 91, 92, 138
decision process 96
Defence, Ministry of *see* Ministry of
  Defence
demand 35, 40, 47, 56, 151, 177, 191
—reduction in 179, 187
demand models *see* models; demand
  relationships 41, 58; demand studies
  43
Department of Employment 5, 122,
  133–138 *passim*, 142, 145, 146–147
—Employment Policy Branch 146
Department of Health and Social
  Security xiii, 82, 83, 85, 88, 113, 122,
  124, 126, 127, 128, 135, 139, 141,
  145, 148
—Health Minister 121, 122
—Secretary of State for Social Services
  88
—ST2 83
Department of the Environment 79
Department of Trade and Industry (DTI)
  5, 85, 86, 122, 124, 133–148 *passim*,
  186–187
—Advisory Panel on Deregulation 143
—Consumer Market Division 141, 145
—Enterprise and Deregulation Unit 85,
  142, 143
—Consumer Safety Unit 144–145
—European Policy Division 144
—General Policy Division 143–144
—International Policy Division 144
—Market Branches 144
—Overseas Trade Divisions 144
—Product Co-ordination Unit 144
—Regional Offices 144
—Secretary of State for Trade and
  Industry 88, 142, 143

Department of Transport 128
department relations 133
departmental-group links 147
departmental interests 122
departmental organisation 136
departmentalism 90, 103, 136
deregulation 142, 147, 173, 175
deregulation units 142
distillation 181
distilled spirit 180
distilleries 139, 180, 182, 183, 185, 186,
  189, 191, 193, 199
—vodka and gin distilleries 200
distillers 85, 121, 125, 159, 161, 163,
  170, 190
Distillers Company 165, 169, 182–187
  passim, 192
distilling 156, 157, 169, 182, 192, 194,
  199, 200, 209, 217, 220, 222
—and rectifying 160
Distilling Sector Working Group 193,
  198
diversification 152, 154, 164, 165, 167,
  170, 172, 177, 183
distribution
—of cigarettes and alcoholic drinks 6,
  88, 140, 183, 210–215 *passim*
distribution networks 151, 165, 192
distributors 179, 204
drinkers 55, 56, 59, 128
—under-age 128
drinking 119, 173, 215
—and driving xiv, 4, 118, 127, 128, 129
—and driving offences 33
—behaviour 51, 59
—domestic drinking habits 139–140
—drunkenness 128
—in public places 119
—legislation 120
—moderate drinking 100
—patterns 147
—policies to reduce drinking 151, 172
—proportion of population 12
drinks, alcohol-free 152
drinks, alcoholic *see* alcoholic drinks
drinks industry *see* alcohol industry
driving offences *see* drinking
drug taking 128
drugs: social science aspects xiii

duty *see also* tax
   see also alcohol
   see also tobacco

EC *see* European Community
ESRC *see* Economic and Social
   Research Council
Early Day Motions *see* Parliamentary
   procedures
EDU *see* Department of Trade and
   Industry. Enterprise and Deregulation
   Unit
economic activity 142
economic adviser 82, 93
economic analysis 3
Economic and Social Research Council
   xii, xiii, xiv
—Exploratory Panel on Addiction xiii
economic conditions 80, 107, 111
economic effects 71
economic factors 1, 19, 72, 133
economic growth 76, 187, 199
economic health 133–134
economic interests 130
economic leverage 123, 124, 126
economic management 106, 108, 136
economic models *see* models
economic objectives 107
economic policy 103, 109, 111
economic power 6
economic rationality 77
economic variables 1, 62
economies of scale 161–162, 165
economy 6, 8, 80, 121, 155, 204, 215,
   216
—local 204
—regional 222
—role of taxes 102
—Scottish 199, 200
—UK 199, 209
education xiv, 136, 137
—alcohol education 130
—health education 32, 100
employment 3, 6, 60, 72, 98, 124, 136,
   156, 157, 163, 179, 191, 192–195,
   204–225
—behaviour 207
—decline in 166
—effects 146, 152, 207, 208, 210, 215,

   216, 222
—geographical distribution 219, 222
—interests 142
—issues 4
—levels of 209, 222
—policy 133, 146, 148
—prospects and opportunities 146, 208,
   224
—trends 208, 209, 220
Employment, Department of *see*
   Department of Employment
Enterprise and Deregulation Unit *see*
   Department of Trade and Industry
Environment, Department of *see*
   Department of the Environment
Europe against Cancer Committee 69, 86
European Community 3, 7, 26, 55,
   65–72 *passim*, 84, 86, 99, 113, 115,
   139, 140, 185
—agricultural levies 84
—directives 139, 140
—harmonisation proposals 102, 69–72
—policies 113
—regulations 32
—Special Wine Working Group 139
—tax harmonisation 3, 26, 55, 66, 86,
   113, 115, 140
—trade policy 144
European Community Commission 70,
   86, 185
European Court 113
European legislation 82, 83
European market 70, 85
Exchequer, Chancellor of *see*
   Chancellor of the Exchequer
excise tax *see* Tax
expenditure
—consumer 2, 9, 10, 11, 13, 33, 215
—government 108
—level of 61
—public expenditure planning 136
—real 9, 10, 11
—relative 11–12
—shares 19
Expenditure Committee *see*
   Parliamentary Select Committees
expenditure series 19, 36
export benefits 176
export policy 139

242

export questions 84
exporters 144
exporting 144
exports 71, 98, 113, 124, 139, 140,
    143–144, 151, 154, 155, 158, 166,
    170, 171, 180, 183, 184, 185, 190,
    195–197, 202, 208

FES *see* Family Expenditure Survey
Faculty of Community Physicians *see*
    Royal College of Physicians
firms *see* companies
fiscal barriers 70
fiscal drag 76
fiscal legislation 70
fiscal measures 143, 208
fiscal policies 75, 82, 92, 100, 103, 115
Fiscal Policy Group *see* HM Treasury
fiscal sovereignty 70
Foreign and Commonwealth Office 86,
    144
Freedom Organisation for the Right to
    Enjoy Smoking Tobacco (FOREST)
    125

GHS *see* General Household Survey
Gallaghers 14, 162, 163, 167, 173, 175
General and Municipal Workers Union
    125
General Household Survey 15, 41, 47
gin *see* alcoholic drinks, spirits
Gin Rectifiers and Distillers Association
    67, 140
Government
—Central 7, 60, 61, 63, 67, 69, 70, 72,
    75–95 *passim*, 99, 103, 104, 108,
    111, 114, 115, 117, 120, 121, 123,
    127, 130, 134, 136, 137, 142, 148,
    151, 159, 180, 205, 206
—Conservative 4, 96, 97, 109, 111, 114,
    121
—departments 96, 123, 127, 135,
    137–147
—Labour 4, 82, 96, 114, 115, 171, 172
—local 135
—machinery of 121–123, 1, 3
—ministers 79
—objectives 92
—policy 3, 102, 121, 128, 155, 173,
    175, 176

—revenue 2, 26, 30–32
—structure of 80–86
—structures 149
Grand Metropolitan 160, 162, 163, 167,
    169
Guinness 154, 159, 161, 162, 163, 165,
    168, 169, 182, 185, 186, 187, 190, 192

HM Customs and Excise xiii, 3, 12, 14,
    28, 30, 67, 75–95 *passim*, 102, 122,
    124, 139, 143, 145
—Assistant Secretary 84
—Customs officials 88, 89, 93, 98
—Departmental Planning Unit 84, 85
—Permanent Secretary 84
—Policy Branch 84
—Revenue Duties Division A 84, 85,
    86, 88, 143, 145
—Tobacco Products Branch 86, 88
—Revenue Duties Division B 84, 85,
    86, 140
—Statistics Branch 84
—King's Beam House 88
HM Treasury 3, 47, 48, 50, 58, 59, 60,
    75–95 *passim*, 97, 98, 100, 103, 122,
    124, 127
—Fiscal Policy Group 81, 82, 83
—Indirect Taxation Division 83
—Public Service Sector 83
Hanson Trust 162, 163, 165, 174
harm 57, 67, 71, 75
—caused by excess use of alcohol 99
—in relation to tar content 56
—levels of 55, 56, 66
—prevention of 104
—smoking 176
Healey, Dennis 4, 82, 106
health 4, 8, 64, 68, 71, 75–76, 88, 92,
    113, 121, 125, 136, 152
—and safety 137
—and smoking 97
—and social services 103
—and welfare issues 103, 136
—education 1, 4, 5, 32, 38, 45, 46–47,
    50, 117, 158, 208, 215; effects of
    health education 46–47, 51
—effects 38, 47, 56, 69, 72, 100, 103,
    104, 109, 142, 148, 179
—expenditure 83

243

—gains 6, 111, 133
—grounds 122, 199
—implications 100, 102, 173
—information programmes 36, 97, 98, 158
—networks 135
—objectives 76, 96, 104, 107, 109, 180
—preventive health objectives 54–74, 103, 117
—policies 58, 61, 63, 65, 69, 71, 72, 114, 126, 174
—risks 32, 56
—shocks 171, 172
—trends 65
—warnings 141, 158, 208
Health and Safety at Work Act 135
Health, Department of see Department of Health and Social Services
Health Education Authority (Council) xiii, 65, 98, 100, 105, 127, 141, 169, 172
Health Minister see Department of Health and Social Services, Health Promotion Research Trust xiii
Home Office xiii, 124, 127, 138, 142, 147, 148
—Criminal Justice and Constitutional Department. Division A. Liquor Licensing Section 147
hotels 139, 163, 164, 165, 212
House of Commons 69, 89
—European Select Committee 82, 83
House of Lords 118, 76
—European Select Committee 75, 82, 83
Howe, Sir Geoffrey 4, 90, 109, 111

IAS see Institute for Alcohol Studies
IDACS see Inter-department advisory committees
ITPAC see Imported Tobacco Products Advisory Council
illness, alcohol-related 179
Imperial Tobacco 145, 156, 162, 163, 165, 167, 169, 173, 174, 175
import penetration 86, 88
Imported Tobacco Products Advisory Council 124, 145
imports 26, 84, 86, 158, 159, 208
income 2, 8, 19, 21, 37, 41–43, 57, 63, 99, 135, 151, 179, 187, 204, 219
—changes 62
—distribution of 219
—elasticity 40, 45–50 passim
—Government 91
—groups 59
—increasing 62, 64
—trends 19–26
    see also Personal Disposable Income
indexation 58, 61, 62, 63, 90, 91, 111, 114
Indirect Taxation Division see HM Treasury. Indirect Taxation Division
industrial competition 66
industrial interests 142
industrial policies 133, 148
industrial sponsorship 90
industrial structure 174
industrialists 207
industry 3, 58, 60, 66, 69, 72, 133
—British 142–144
—network 135
—performance 166–173
    see also alcohol industry, Scotch whisky industry, tobacco industry
inflation 61, 62, 66, 90, 91, 98, 107, 109, 112, 113, 114, 158, 159
information, role of xiv
information system 205–206
Inland Revenue 81
Institute for Alcohol Studies xiii, 127
Interdepartment advisory committees (IDACS) 137
interdepartmental coordination 136, 137, 138
interdepartmental conflict 122, 123
interdepartmental discussions 124
interest groups 79, 151, 155, 171, 175
—producer interest groups 152
    see also lobbies, pressure groups

job-displacing effects 206
job losses 6, 98, 151, 171, 200, 204–224 passim
—by location 219–222
jobs 6, 155, 176
—dependent on alcohol and tobacco production 210–216

labelling, food and drink 141
labour *see* work force
Labour administration 96, 114
Labour Party 121
—manifesto 120
—policy 120
labour requirements 215, 216
lager *see* alcoholic drinks, beer
Lawson, Nigel 4, 78, 82, 98, 111
legislation 61, 69, 108, 120, 135, 155
—on smoking 122
  see also fiscal legislation
liberalisation 173, 175
Licensed House Managers and Tenants
  101
licensed premises
  see also public houses 39, 48, 49, 50,
164, 205
licensed production 160
licensing 48, 49, 142, 165
—boards 38–39, 119
—hours 120, 146
—laws 38–39, 120, 122, 147, 171, 172,
  175, 205
—changes in Scottish licensing laws 39
—liquor xiv, 119, 124, 146
Licensing Act (Scotland) 1976 147
lobbies 118, 123, 128, 130, 155, 168,
  176, 177, 180, 189, 208
—alcohol industry 89, 97, 100, 101,
  123, 125
—health 3, 4–7, 35, 58, 67, 75, 96–103,
  106, 109, 111, 114, 115, 123–130
  passim, 133, 145
—industrial 123–126, 111
—Scotch whisky 133, 114, 115
—Scottish 192
—tobacco trade 58, 89, 97, 99, 123, 125
—trade 1, 4–6, 35, 72, 89, 96–100, 106,
  109, 111, 113, 114, 115, 121, 123
—wine 71
  see also pressure groups, interest
groups
lobby criticism 111
lobby influence 4, 5, 177
lobby opinion 96
lobby pressure 111, 113
lobbying 78, 88, 89, 100, 146, 147, 151

MAFF *see* Ministry of Agriculture,
  Fisheries and Food
MPs *see* politicians
macroeconomic level 87
macroeconomic objectives 61, 72
macroeconomic policy 76, 81, 93, 114
macroeconomic purposes 4
malt 180
—distilling capacity 190
—distilling process 192
—Campbeltown 181
—Dundee 181
—Greenock 181
—Highland 181
—Lowland 181, 182
—vatted 181
—whisky 196
malting 156, 157, 160, 193, 209, 210,
  217, 220
manufacturers' costs *see* costs
manufacturing base 151
manufacturing industry 156, 157, 209,
  217, 219, 220
—employment in 210, 214, 222
market changes 62
market environment 176
market forces 43
market opportunities 159, 161
market shares 11, 159, 190, 197, 199
—of beer 32
—of spirits 32
—relative 32
market trends 158
marketing 153, 154, 174, 189, 192, 195
markets 1, 7, 161, 165, 173, 175, 187,
  196, 208
—export 156, 158, 172, 182, 183, 190,
  196, 198, 199, 202
—European 71
—home 71, 156, 158, 162, 172,
  182–202 *passim*, 210, 215
—import 159
—international 80, 187, 210, 215
—labour 208, 215
—whisky 186
  see also alcohol markets
  see also tobacco markets
maturation 181, 182, 193
media 123, 137, 145

—influence of public opinion on 129
media opinion 117
media pressure 119
mergers and take-overs 152, 153, 161, 162, 164, 165–166, 170, 172, 175, 182, 185, 187, 210, 5
minimum drinking age 39
Minister for Agriculture *see* Ministry of Agriculture, Fisheries and Food
Ministerial Group on Alcohol Misuse 138, 141, 148
Ministry of Agriculture, Fisheries and Food (MAFF) 5, 85, 86, 88, 122, 124, 133–148 *passim*
—Alcoholic Drinks Division 139, 140
—Cereals Division 139
—Food Science Division 139
—Horticultural Division 139
—Standards Division 139, 141
Minister for Agriculture 88
Ministry of Defence 79
Ministry of Labour 146
models 2, 35–53, 208
—administrative constraints model 77, 80, 92
—clientella models 147
—demand models 35, 39–43, 50, 51, 64
—economic models 79, 207
—employment and unemployment models 205
—monopoly models 153
—partial adjustment model 43
—perfect competition models 153
—single-equation models 41–42
—statistical models 40, 171–173
—structure-performance models 152, 153, 176
—theoretical models 41–42
Monopolies and Mergers Commission 174, 175, 183, 186, 192, 143
monopolies 152, 153, 161, 165, 169, 173, 174
—policy 175
—state 66
—economic models: monopoly *see* models
multiplier 6
—employment 200, 203, 213, 214
networks 137, 138, 148, 168

see also organisational networks, policy networks, producer network, industry network, health network
—inter-network coordination 138
—network boundaries 137

off-licensed trade 185
off-licences 164, 211, 213
oligopoly 153, 173, 174
opinion *see* public opinion, parliamentary opinion, media opinion
organisation by services 136
organisational networks 134, 135, 137, 148
organisational parochialism 4
organisational structures 138, 148
output 153–175 *passim*, 200, 201, 202, 206–216 *passim*
ownership 5, 167, 168, 169, 172, 180, 185, 189, 190

PDI *see* Personal Disposable Income
PESC *see* Public Expenditure Survey Committee
PSBR *see* Public Sector Borrowing Requirement
Parliament 4, 63, 69, 89, 97, 101, 102, 115, 118, 119, 120, 130, 180
Parliamentary Alcohol Policy and Services Group 118
Parliamentary Expenditure Committee *see* Parliamentary Select Committees
parliamentary opinion 96, 97, 101, 103, 114, 118
parliamentary procedures
—Early Day Motions 101, 103, 104
—Adjournment Debates 101, 103
—Parliamentary Motions 104
—Parliamentary Questions 4, 101–103, 118
Parliamentary Select Committees 83, 75
—Expenditure Committee 75, 97
parliamentary support 101–104, 120
passive smoking
see smoking, passive
paternalism 3
paternalist policies 57, 61
penalties for drink-driving offences 129
performance *see* industry performance

perry *see* alcoholic drinks
Personal Disposable Income (PDI) 20, 21, 37, 47
pipe tobacco 15, 17, 42, 113, 156
—consumption of 69
pluralism 77–78, 79, 87, 92
policies *see* economic policies; employment policies; fiscal policies; Government policies; industrial policies; prevention policies
policy
—advisers 91, 93, 121
—analysts 75
—changes 39, 117, 158, 207
—choice 80
—coordination 137
—debates 39
—developments 143, 146
—effect of 4, 41
—formation 1, 3, 4, 50, 51, 134, 135, 137
—implementation 134, 135, 137
—innovation 76
—instrument 37, 70
—issues 122, 123, 137, 173
—makers 123, 130, 135, 152, 155, 172, 179, 205, 208
—making 78, 80–93, 124, 148
—networks 134
—objectives 3
—options 78, 105
—process 475–95, 135, 148: theoretical perspectives 77–80
—proposals 143, 146
—recommendations 83
—relevance 36
—statements 97
—structure 75–95
political advisors 81
political change 96
political environment 117, 123
political factors 72
political objectives 107
political obstacles 117
political parties 117, 120, 123
political power 6, 80
political science 79, 117
political support 71, 79
political system (British) 4, 134

political variables 1
politicians 4, 7, 118, 79, 91, 118–120, 123, 155
—local 117, 119, 120, 121
—MPs 4, 89, 99, 102, 103, 118, 120, 123, 127, 146; backbench MPs 101, 103, 104, 118, 120; Conservative MPs 78, 103, 135; Labour MPs 99
—national 117, 118, 119, 120
—Assistant Secretary 143
—Ministers 80, 81, 87, 119, 121, 122, 136, 138, 147
—Prime Minister 70, 81, 82, 88, 89
—Principal Secretary 143
—Under Secretary 143
politics
—domestic 143
—economic 143
—financial 143
—fiscal 143
—of confrontation 5
—of prevention 117–132
—Party politics 120–121
population 2, 15, 33
population size 36
—smoking population 18
pressure groups 77, 78, 79, 83, 89, 92, 97, 100, 117, 118, 123–135, 176
see also interest groups; lobbies
prevention 5, 55, 69, 90, 91, 104, 208
—impediments to 138
—in relation to health 54–74, 117
—politics of 117–132
—strategy of 66, 69, 133, 147, 215
prevention measures 152, 155, 205, 208
prevention policy 1, 5, 6, 26, 36, 40–45 *passim*, 50, 86, 93, 97, 100, 103, 114, 118, 121, 129, 149–158 *passim*, 161, 168, 170–177 *passim*, 179–203, 204–224 *passim*
prices 1, 2, 8, 21, 41, 42, 43, 58, 63, 66, 69, 108, 109, 151, 152, 161, 173
—and income 37, 57
—changes 58, 63, 64, 106, 107, 112
—control 75, 92
—cross price effects 37
—deflators 37
—elasticity 40, 45, 47, 48, 49, 50, 58, 60
—increase in 57, 61, 62, 64, 108, 151,

153, 205
—index 19, 20, 63
—levels 58, 61, 62, 75, 82
—movement in 111
—notifications 66
—real own 37, 62, 64, 69, 75
—regulation xiv
—relative 19, 32, 37, 72, 159
—retail 110, 112, 198
—trends 2, 18, 19–26
—variations 19, 40, 47, 100
Prime Minister *see* politicians
Prime Minister's Policy Unit 82, 89, 93
producer groups 114, 133, 135, 155,
    173, 175, 176, 177, 205
producer interests 4, 5, 135
producer network 135, 137, 138, 139
Producer Price Index 160
producers 1, 6, 7, 151, 176, 179, 187,
    199, 204, 208
—government/producer relations 133,
    134
product shares 12
production 136, 148, 189, 199, 215
production facilities (overseas) 183
production network 137
production process 180–182, 219
productivity 152, 166, 171
profitability 5, 6, 151, 152, 154,
    161–177 *passim*
profits 1, 5, 124, 125, 153, 163, 165,
    171–173, 177
—manufacturers' profits 64
public attitudes 4
public awareness 100
public bodies 83
public choice 204
—public choice analysis 176
—public choice theory 79
public concern 176
public debates 9, 87
public education campaigns 32
public expenditure 76, 79, 82, 83, 87,
    89, 91, 92, 103
Public Expenditure Survey Committee
    137
public health 5, 80, 89, 92, 101–104,
    117, 176
public health campaigners 89, 92

public houses 39, 139, 151, 204, 211,
    212, 215
—tied-houses 140, 156, 164, 165, 174,
    175, 185
see also licensed premises
public image 129
public interest 12, 153, 174–176
public objectives 76, 77
public opinion xiv, 4, 63, 66, 89, 96, 97,
    99, 100, 104–105, 114, 117, 128, 130
public order 147, 152, 176
public policy 3, 89, 90, 173–176
public relations 155, 176
Public Sector Borrowing Requirement
    108, 109
Public Service Sector
    see HM Treasury
public support 97, 104, 120, 128, 130
purchasing power 1, 2, 19, 21, 26, 32

RCP *see* Royal College of Physicians
RDA *see* HM Customs and Excise.
    Revenue Duties Division A
RDB *see* HM Customs and Excise.
    Revenue Duties Division B
ROSPA *see* Royal Society for the
    Prevention of Accidents
RPI *see* Retail Price Index
regulation 36, 38–39, 80, 85, 142, 143,
    176
regulator 108
regulatory policies 152
relative prices *see* prices, relative
restaurants 139, 163, 165, 211, 212
Retail Price Index 9, 19, 20, 37, 62, 63,
    65, 89, 103, 106, 108, 110, 112, 157,
    160, 201, 220
retail outlets 154, 161, 164, 165
retailers
—alcoholic drinks and cigarettes 88, 151
—tobacco 155
retailing 174, 210–215 *passim*, 224
retailing associations 211
retailing issues 140
revalorisation 3, 61–63, 66, 72, 91, 108
revenue *see* taxation revenue
Revenue Divisions *see* HM Customs and
    Excise
Rothmans 145, 156, 162, 163, 167, 175

Royal College of General Practitioners 126

Royal College of Physicians 38, 46, 47, 97, 126, 127, 128, 158, 171

—Faculty of Community Physicians 126

Royal College of Psychiatrists 65, 126, 128

Royal Colleges of Medicine 126, 127, 128

Royal Society for the Prevention of Accidents 127

SIC *see* Standard Industrial Classification

safety

—on roads 179

safety interests *see* consumer interests

salaries *see* wages

sales 1, 6, 154, 158, 166, 167, 170, 173, 174, 196, 198, 219

—overseas 6, 162

sales promotion 183

Scotch Whisky Association 23, 67, 88, 100, 124, 140, 191, 198, 184

Scotch whisky industry 4, 6, 56, 101, 111, 113, 114, 115, 152, 155, 179–203

—demand 183

—employment trends 192–195

—export trends 195–197

—production trends 190–192

—reactions to prevention policy 198–202

—reduction in demand 180

—sales 182

—taxation policy 198

Scotland 119, 180

—economy of 180, 199, 200

—employment in 6, 219, 220, 222

—political position 115

Scottish and Newcastle 162, 163, 167, 169, 183

Secretary of State for Social Services *see* Department of Health

Secretary of State for Trade and Industry *see* Department of Trade and Industry

'elect Committees *see* Parliamentary Select Committees

Selective Employment Tax *see* Tax, Selective Employment

shareholders 5, 152, 154, 166, 168, 172, 204, 205

shops (stores) 151, 164, 204, 213

smoke-free zones 120

smokers 2, 15, 18, 55, 59, 104, 128

—ex-smokers 104

—men 2, 18, 47

—women 2, 18, 47

smoking 57, 109, 119, 120, 126, 128, 165, 173, 176, 188

—and health 97, 104, 126

—at work 135

—behaviour 51, 59

—effects of 158

—giving up 18

—in public places 128

—in the UK 129

—passive smoking 56

—policies 119, 151, 172

—problems 83, 128

—risks 122, 171

—social and economic costs of 97

—trends in 83

snuff 156

social aspects of smoking and drinking 173

social cost of smoking and drinking xiii, 55, 59, 93

soft drinks 157, 163, 165

—mineral water 156

—fruit and vegetable juices 156

spirits *see* alcoholic drinks

sponsorship 138, 142, 147, 148, 149, 174

—sports sponsorship xiv, 38, 129

Standard Industrial Classification (SIC) 156

Standing Conference on Crime Prevention: Working Group 141

statistical analysis 40

statistical criteria 41, 44

statistical methods 36

statistical models *see* models

statistics 8, 19

structure-performance model *see* models

supermarkets 151, 164, 175, 185, 213, 215

suppliers 151, 154, 155, 174

—foreign 158, 159, 205

—wholesale 182

supplies 136
supply 7, 151, 177
supplying industries 200, 202, 204, 210, 215

TAC *see* Tobacco Advisory Council
TV advertising *see* advertising
tariff barriers 139, 182, 199
tax
—authorities 76, 80, 89
—avoidance of 87
—bands 61–66, 68
—collection of 81, 83, 86, 88, 89, 91, 93, 102, 115
—deferment of 102
—earmarking 90, 91
—elasticity 58, 84
—exemptions 155
—increases 45, 49, 75, 76, 102, 113, 122, 151, 152, 158, 171, 172, 176, 202, 205, 206, 208, 210, 211
—objectives 61, 63, 96, 107, 113
—payers 80
—proposals 80, 87
—proportion 26, 107
—regulations 77
—structures 80, 98
—system 76, 80, 91, 93
—yield 2, 3, 4, 30, 31, 32, 57, 58, 71, 76, 84, 109, 113, 114, 154, 171, 172, 200, 201
taxation 2, 8, 26, 72, 97, 122, 152, 171, 172, 173, 211, 218
—changes in 26, 50, 54, 57–58, 61, 63, 64, 65, 66–69, 76, 84, 87, 89, 99, 106, 107, 108, 112
—commodity 70, 76
—decisions 96
—differential 66–68
—direct 83, 97, 109, 111
—effects of 36, 158
—equalizing of 71
—indirect 26, 76, 82, 83, 84, 91, 97, 109, 111, 124
—levels of 54, 55, 62, 65, 71, 72, 89, 91, 101, 104, 105, 113
—policies 2, 3, 4, 26, 32, 36, 54–74, 75–95, 96–116, 133, 143, 152, 159, 198

—per unit of alcohol 56
—preventive 55, 56, 97
—rates of 4, 32, 37, 55, 57, 58, 62, 63, 64, 70, 77, 99, 100, 104, 106, 109, 110, 111, 113, 114
—real rates 3, 64
—reduction in 88
—specific 69, 84
—structure of 71; alternative taxation structures 66–69
—trends 2, 8–34
—used for control of consumption 100
see also tobacco taxation
taxation revenue 4, 8, 26, 30, 54, 57–61, 62, 72, 102–104, 108, 111, 113, 115, 122, 124, 133
—from alcoholic drink 30, 31, 105
—from tobacco 30, 31, 105
—loss of 111
—revenue departments 122
—revenue management 106
—revenue requirements 76, 80, 89, 91
—source of revenue 30, 54, 55, 60–61
taxes
—ad valorem 26, 28, 66, 67, 69, 71, 106
—company 70
—corporation 198
—customs duty 84
—excise 14, 26, 27, 29, 60, 62, 66, 67, 70, 76, 80, 84, 86, 90, 91, 98, 108, 110–113, 114, 143, 158, 159, 180, 198
—expenditure 30, 31, 32
—general sales 60, 70
—import duty 26, 140
—income 70, 91
—retail price 198
—selective employment 87
—tobacco leaf duty 26, 27, 28
—tobacco product duty 28, 66
—VAT 26, 28, 31, 60, 62, 67, 69, 70, 76, 84, 85, 87, 107, 108, 110, 181, 198
—wealth tax 87
—wine duty 26–27
technical change 207, 218
technical issues 85
technical progress 166, 210
technological factors 62

technology 206, 20, 217, 219, 224
temperance organisations 127
tied-houses *see* public houses
time-series data, analysis 9, 41, 194, 219
time-series study 173
tobacco 8, 11, 15, 19, 42, 45–47, 50, 60,
    62, 64, 65, 68, 70, 72, 75, 76, 85,
    108, 117, 118, 121, 126, 155, 156,
    157, 160, 163, 164, 176
—chewing 28
—demand for 35, 36, 38, 44, 176, 215
—expenditure on 9, 10, 11, 13
—handrolling 15, 17, 28
—leaf 26
—markets, marketing 1, 2, 6, 15, 32, 83,
    145, 151, 152, 154
—policy 119, 123, 128, 134, 147, 173
—prices 2, 19, 20, 54, 63, 66, 86, 93,
    109
—producers 88, 134, 141, 149, 156, 159
—production 6, 118, 154
—products 2, 151, 152, 177, 205
—retailing of 39
—revenue from sales 5, 6, 204, 213
—tar content 56
—trade 98, 99, 102
—use 3, 4, 7, 9, 32, 124, 129, 130
—weight 15, 17, 36, 56
Tobacco Advisory Council 17, 34, 47,
    88, 98, 124, 125, 145, 176, 211
Tobacco Alliance 99
tobacco consumption 1, 8, 9, 15, 17, 18,
    32, 35, 37, 41–47 *passim*, 50, 56, 64,
    75, 83, 93, 97, 109, 115, 126, 224
—decrease in 15, 65, 75, 122
—health implications 97, 124, 147
—health issues 120, 121, 124, 126, 127
—problems associated with 103, 117,
    122, 129
—tobacco-related harm 104
tobacco industry 1, 5, 6, 8, 76, 86, 88,
    89, 101, 102, 118, 120–121, 122–127
    passim, 133, 138, 141–146 *passim*,
    151–178, 204–225
—employment in 210
—factories 85
—manufacturing interests 145
—women in 6
—workers 205

tobacco leaf duty *see* taxes
tobacco taxation 4, 26, 27, 30, 31, 32,
    58–61, 65, 69, 71, 76, 96, 99, 101,
    104–105, 106, 108, 109, 111, 115,
    122, 145
—changes in 97
—duty 65, 60–70, 76, 77, 83–86, 89,
    91–93, 97, 103, 109, 111, 113, 114,
    143
—economic role of 102
—freeze in 99
—increases in 99, 108, 111, 113, 128
—policy 54–74, 104
—rates 97
—revenue from 113
Tobacco Workers Union 125
tobacconists 211, 212
trade
—balance of 60
—barriers to 86
—effects of tax policy on 3
Trade and Industry, Department of *see*
    Department of Trade and Industry
trade agreements 144
trade associations 83, 87, 140, 141, 145,
    155, 176, 205, 211
trade fairs 144
trade interests 83, 84
trade missions 144
Trade Unions 125, 205, 206, 207, 219
Transport and General Workers Union
    125
transport 204
Transport, Ministry of *see* Ministry of
    Transport
Treasury *see* HM Treasury
trends *see* taxation trends; consumption
    trends; price and income trends

unemployment 158, 204, 207, 208, 224
—high levels of 107, 216
—low levels of 108
—redundancies 199, 200
unemployment areas 6, 211, 220, 222
unemployment rates 6, 199, 205
United Kingdom Accounts *see* Central
    Statistical Office
VAT *see* Tax
variables 36–39, 40, 48

variation in prices *see* prices, variations
   in
vodka *see* alcoholic drinks, spirits

WHO *see* World Health Organisation
wages 219, 220
—rates 206
—levels 206, 208
whisky *see* alcoholic drinks
Whitbread 129, 162, 163, 167, 168, 169,
   186
Whitehall 3, 5, 78, 81, 119, 122, 127,
   128, 142
wine *see* alcoholic drinks
Wine and Spirits Liaison Committee 118
Wines and Spirits Association 124, 140
work force 98, 154, 191, 192, 200, 206,
219, 222
workers 6, 204, 207, 208
—female 21–26, 216–219 *passim*, 224
—full-time 205, 211, 216
—low-paid 219
—male 21–26, 217–218, 224
—manual 21–26
—part-time 205, 208, 216
—skilled 205, 206, 216
—unskilled 206, 208, 216
working days lost 179
working parties
World Health Organisation 65
—Collaborating Centre for Research
   and Training in the Psychosocial and
   Economic Aspects of Health xiii